AF880620

HEALTH SERVICES ADMINISTRATION:
Education and Practice

HEALTH SERVICES ADMINISTRATION:
Education and Practice

by

KAREN M. LORENTZEN, R.N., Ed.D.
Professor and Chairperson
Department of Health
University of Lowell
Lowell, Massachusetts

LINDA ROEMER, Ph.D.
Assistant Professor, Department of Health
Graduate Coordinator
Program in Health Services Administration
University of Lowell
Lowell, Massachusetts

WARREN H. GREEN, INC.
St. Louis, Missouri, U.S.A.

Published by

WARREN H. GREEN, INC.
8356 Olive Boulevard
St. Louis, Missouri 63132, U.S.A.

All rights reserved

©1988 by WARREN H. GREEN, INC.

ISBN No. 0-87527-353-X

Printed in the United States of America

Introduction

Health Services Administration is a broad-based discipline with practitioners from divergent educational and occupational backgrounds. The authors believe that Health Services Administration, as an emerging and growing profession, needs to emphasize, even demand, professional preparation on the college and university level. These preparatory programs emphasize skills and knowledge related to the profession as well as training in the health sciences and liberal arts.

If the primary goal of education is achievement of specified outcomes by learners — skills, knowledge, and attitudes — then educators must accept the role of manager of the learning process. Through effective preparatory programs, led by strong educators, the profession of Health Services Administration will be nurtured, enhanced, and strengthened.

The authors, who educate students to be administrators of health services, have identified the need to define the field more clearly, particularly in relation to education. In addition, there is a need for a single pragmatic resource containing information of significance to students, educators, and practitioners of Health Services Administration. Ideally, this book will serve as a reference for students and practitioners and as a contemporary resource for educators in the field. It has been designed to meet these needs by gathering and organizing essential information into a compact and convenient form.

Acknowledgments

The authors wish to thank the following individuals who provided support and encouragement during the development of this book. Carl Lorentzen, Michael Roemer, Beverly Volicer, and Mark Synderman made helpful comments on the manuscript. Sally Healey and Jeanne Kaloustian gave freely of their time and efforts while typing the drafts of the manuscript. Our thanks to Eleanor Shalhoup for helping us to clarify our view of Health Services Administration.

Karen M. Lorentzen, R.N., Ed.D.
Linda Roemer, Ph.D.

University of Lowell
Lowell, Massachusetts

Contents

HEALTH SERVICES ADMINISTRATION:
Education and Practice

Chapter 1

The Historical Development

The primary purpose of any health care system is to achieve an optimal level of health for a specific population. Health services can be defined as all personal and public services provided by institutions or individuals for the purpose of maintaining or restoring health (1).

A health care system is an organized, planned effort — at the community, state, or national level — to attain a set of pre-established health goals through the provision of health services (2). Viewing health services as part of a system facilitates planning and delivery of these services within the context of a total societal environment. Public and private organizations, in a variety of complex configurations and subsystems, provide the health care services that are used.

The ultimate purpose of the health care system is the delivery of health care services to the people who need them. The planned and organized delivery of comprehensive health care services, provided in a manner satisfactory to the consumer, should be the prime concern of the system and those who administer it.

The health care system in the United States is growing and undergoing dramatic change. While scientific discoveries and technological advances make services more complex and expansive, there is greater demand for more health care as well as containment of the costs of that health care. Policy makers and academics debate the distribution of funds between highly technological services, such as organ transplants or coronary bypass surgery, and more basic services, such as home care for the elderly. While this debate goes on, pragmatic resource allocation decisions are made daily by health professionals.

At the same time that the system has become more complex, the environment within which the health care system operates has changed. Regulatory, financial, political, and social changes have greatly affected the health care system. Reflection on external and internal changes leads to the conclusion that both medically and organizationally, the health care system is very different now than it was just a decade ago. It seems likely that change will continue at the same or an accelerated pace.

The individuals who plan and manage health care services are health services administrators. Health Services Administration is a unique discipline, with its own body of knowledge, which incorporates and integrates knowledge from other disciplines such as management and the behavioral or social sciences. Health Services is a process, not isolated acts or decisions.

The complex and changing health care system requires administrators with broad views and specialized knowledge, skills, and competencies. Education can provide practitioners and potential practitioners with the opportunity to acquire these skills, instill professional attitudes, and give students, through field placements, an opportunity to practice the competencies necessary for effective administration.

The last century has seen major changes within the American health care system. These have been brought about as a result of major changes in the health needs of the population it serves, the technology available, and the delivery and administration of those health services. The primary health problems within our system have changed from epidemics of acute infections to chronic illnesses, with all the complexities, demands, difficulties, and long-term concerns associated with these conditions. There was little technology available in the mid-nineteenth century; today, there is abundant and rapidly increasing technology. This has posed problems for the health services administrator, the manager of the system, who is forced to balance resources and needs.

In today's society, social values and priorities have altered dramatically. From an approach in the nineteenth century that relied on individual or charitable assistance, the pendulum has swung so that society now holds health care as a right and views the guarantee of that right as government's responsibility, as demonstrated by the passage of Medicare and Medicaid.

These changes are reflected in the history and development of Health Services Administration which is closely associated with and connected to the history and development of hospital administration. From the founding of the Pennsylvania Hospital in 1752 until the end of the nineteenth century, hospital administration was not seen as a specialized field of endeavor.

By the beginning of the twentieth century it was recognized that special training was necessary to run a hospital. A great deal of the training for these positions took place on the job, and these positions traditionally were filled by nurses or doctors, referred to as superintendents, whose primary responsibility was the maintenance and supervision of supplies, property, and equipment. Individuals interested in training for such a position assumed an apprenticeship under the superintendent (3).

In the late 1920s, Michael Davis at the University of Chicago offered a new concept — that hospital administration was a career. In 1932, this was reinforced by the Committee on the Costs of Medical Care which stated that hospitals and clinics were social and business enterprises that should be under the direction of trained and prepared health services administrators.

In the early 1930s, Davis developed the first course in hospital administration. It was incorporated into a graduate program offering a Master of Business Administration degree. The program included course work and a year-long administrative residency off-campus at a selected hospital (5).

It is interesting to note some of the important events in the development of the field of Health Services Administration:

1929 —Michael Davis, publication of *Hospital Administration: A Career.*

1933 —American College of Hospital Administration founded.

1934 —Michael Davis, University of Chicago, established the first course in Health Administration, a course in the Graduate School of Business Administration.

1945 —A Joint Commission on Education examined the educational requirements for entry into Health Administration. From this Commission evolved a core curriculum for Health Administration programs addressing the areas of: the medical staff, personnel management, medical care programs, business and financial management, community relations.

1948 —Formation of the national association of these programs, Association of University Programs in Hospital Administration (now Health Administration), AUPHA.

1954 —The Commission on University Education in Hospital Administration implemented an educational study for future programs in hospital administration and a review of existing programs. The recommendations of the Commission were:

1) A joining of liberal arts education with professional and operational aspects of administration.
2) Foundation courses: mathematics and statistics, psychology, sociology, economics.
3) Functional fields were identified as: finance, marketing, and personnel (6).

The Commission stated that a program of studies should address five main concepts:

1. Information on organization and management of hospitals.
2. Proficiency in exploration and solution of problems in addition to decision making in the area of administration.
3. Efficient communication and effective handling of people, individually and collectively.
4. Complete understanding of the current economic and social system in which hospitals function and individuals live.
5. Inquiring mind, independent thinking, and emotional maturity (7).

Included in this report were recommendations for faculty standards, program functioning within a university setting, and qualifications for the program director (8).

1972 through 1974 — A study of health administrators was conducted under the auspices of the W.K. Kellogg Foundation and addressed education as it related to contemporary health services delivery problems. The Commission's findings directly affected and had great significance for the future of health administration. The report was titled, *Education for Health Administration* (12), and some of the findings of the Commission were not only informative but surprising:

1) The need to educate new and current practitioners. Less than 25% of executive positions were filled by personnel with formal health administration training.
2) The need for continuing education to maintain ongoing competence for practicing administrators.
3) Programs of study must be strengthened to prepare students for leadership roles. Health administrative programs must include course work in health topics, management, and administration, with greater coordination between didactic work and field experience.

4) The quality of education can be improved by increasing faculty size, visibility of programs, and affiliation with health practice.
5) The pool of program applicants should be increased to improve student quality and recruitment.
6) Collaboration with other disciplines and an interdisciplinary approach should be emphasized (9).

Detailing these events clearly shows the subtle transformation of the profession that is recognized today as Health Services Administration.

Changes in the educational approach and process reflect shifts in the role, title, duties, functions, and responsibilities the health service administrator has experienced over the past fifty years (10). The hospital superintendent of fifty years ago, who was not specifically trained and educated for this managerial position, is now acknowledged as the Chief Executive Officer, Administrator, President, Director, or has a similar administrative title and ideally is prepared and educated in a carefully-developed program.

This contemporary administrator may be a member of a wide variety of professional organizations, hold a baccalaureate, master's, or doctoral degree in the specialty, and direct the total operation of a large and complex hospital, long-term care facility, community agency, or related health organization.

Health care is characterized by change in virtually every area of operation. In this dynamic milieu the health services administrator is confronted with changing financial requirements, quality control and assurance, organizational arrangements, new mergers, government regulation, changing consumer demands, and other shifts in the environment. The demands and expectations are great, the related professional evolution in this century has been dramatic, the future is exciting and challenging.

The health administrator is subjected to a complex set of demands which are frequently in opposition or competition with one another. Administrators must constantly seek to develop and maintain proper perspective between means and ends (11), between organizational needs and the expanded community view. In order to accomplish this, the health administrator must be a facilitator of the public interest within the organization and the community; this requires a professional with a high degree of administrative creativity, flexibility, and change of orientation (12).

REFERENCES

1. Levey and Loomba, *Health Care Administration*, p. 4
2. *Ibid.*
3. Bellin and Weeks, *The Challenge of Administering Health Services*, p. 15.
4. *Ibid.*
5. *Ibid.*
6. *Ibid.*
7. *Ibid.*, pp. 15-16.
8. *Ibid.*
9. *Education for Health Administration.*
10. Bellin and Weeks, p. 17.
11. *Education for Health Administration*, p. 147
12. *Ibid.*

Chapter 2

Issues and Trends

Health services administrators face a number of pressures, many of them conflicting. The health services administrator is often caught in the middle, balancing available resources against need and demand for health services. Many of these trends and issues seem likely to persist into the future, continuing to strongly affect the ways in which health services are administered.

Cost containment is primary in importance as national health policy, despite the increased demand for services generated by the rise in the elderly population. Health promotion competes with new technology and research for scarce dollars.

There has been considerable aggregation of health care facilities and agencies, with many organizations integrating horizontally and vertically. Health services administrators develop, work within, or respond to changing types of organizational structures within the health care system. Health Maintenance Organizations (HMO) development, at least on the grand scale of the past, may have peaked, but variations such as Preferred Provider Organizations are of increasing interest. New forms of multi–institutional arrangements are being developed and tried.

Health care organizations face internal changes as well. Cost containment pressures require more fiscal accountability with leaner, tighter organizations. The use of computerized management information systems (MIS) continues to grow and expand into patient care. Health services administrators are required to be more specialized. Materials management, patient accounts, marketing, reimbursement, and scheduling increasingly are being handled by specialists, at least in large organizations.

Regulatory and reimbursement structures and systems are also changing. The placing of caps on capital expenditures for acute care is an important thrust. Despite continual efforts to eliminate them, Health Systems Agencies are thriving in some parts of the country. Even where they have been eliminated there have been efforts to contain costs, particularly those associated with new services or facilities.

Payors and reimbursers are seeking to reduce their expenses, leaving administrators to spend large amounts of time lobbying and negotiating for fair rates of payment which will enable them to service those who are in need.

COST CONTAINMENT AND ACCESS

Cost containment has dominated and will continue to dominate national health policy and to be the major influence on most health care organizations. Resources are finite and the changing age structure of the United States' population guarantees increasing demands. People live longer and die frailer, and with less family support than in the past. This guarantees increasing demand for services at all levels of the health care system, from home care to acute-care hospitals.

These cost containment pressures require health services administrators to run efficient and effective organizations. There is less room for inefficiencies. Third-party payors extract increasing compliance to efficiency standards as the price of survival.

Health services administrators are on the firing line in the battles between cost containment and access. It is administrators, not policy makers, who in the last analysis make decisions about how scarce resources are distributed and who is denied services. Administrators, particularly in inner cities, rural areas, and in areas of the country that are hard hit by declining industry, are under pressure to provide services for which there is no payment.

Lower cost hospitals, particularly in urban areas, are more likely to close than others, leaving residents of inner city areas, particularly minority members, without adequate care or forcing them to leave the cities to go to more expensive care elsewhere (1). This pattern affects other areas of the health care system as well. There are, not surprisingly, far fewer nursing home beds in areas with large minority populations. As the cost of keeping Medicaid patients in nursing homes rises, as it inevitably must, two things happen. First, efforts are made to prevent, or to put off as long as possible, nursing home admissions. This is a good thing, as long as adequate support services are available to maintain independent living in the community. Second, nursing homes, and the administrators who run them, are likely to come under considerable criticism for their allegedly profligate ways, just as administrators in acute-care settings are partially blamed for rising costs. While criticism of rates which seem unconscionably low to a nursing administrator may seem absurd, those outside of the field find it difficult to accept the true cost of nursing home care.

Similar pressures exist in mental health. The costs and difficulties associated with supplying comprehensive, integrated, community-based care have not been adequately calculated nor described. They are likely to be considerably higher than the cost of providing care in state mental hospitals. While this has long been admitted by those in the field, policy makers and those who have to vote state and federal support have not fully accepted community-based programs which are also more diffuse and, therefore, harder to hold accountable. There is, therefore, increasing pressure on community-based programs, even before they are established at minimum standards (2).

Although industry has developed alcohol treatment programs for employees, most substance abusers face decreasing sympathy from those who pay, and there may be a return to viewing the abuser as responsible, morally and financially, for his or her problem. Administrators find increasing resistance to the establishment of programs for those whom it is thought could help themselves, if they would only try.

Administrators of nonprofit health care organizations face increasingly difficult moral issues. Efficiency and economies of scale go only so far. At some point, administrators have to refuse services to some people in order to save their organizations. Reimbursement systems such as Ch. 372 in Massachusetts aggravate the situation by increasing the incentive to take private pay or Blue Cross patients over Medicaid and free care or charity patients. As the for-profit sector of the system expands, a smaller number of nonprofit organizations are left to absorb those who cannot pay.

Where there is excess in the system, as in older cities in the East and Midwest, such incentives are partially balanced by organizational needs to maintain operating levels. Where beds and services are in short supply, there is little financial incentive to care for patients who do not have insurance or cannot pay for themselves. The United States appears to have accelerated in the direction of a two-class system of health care, and increasing numbers of Americans are not able to obtain health care. Those in the middle as this situation becomes worse are health services administrators.

REGULATION AND COMPETITION

Cost pressures have led to increased regulation. Despite philosophical and practical difficulties in implementation, it seems likely that regulation will continue to be used to contain costs.

Increasing costs and the realization by industry and labor that ultimately they bear these costs, led to increased demand for control and regulation of health care. The federal government, which in 1981 paid $.29 of every dollar spent on health care (3), has taken the lead in attempting to control costs, in part by instituting prospective payment by Diagnostically Related Groups (DRGs).

Two areas of cost are receiving particular attention. The first is capital expenditure, particularly the large amounts required to renovate and modernize the physical plants of older, acute-care hospitals. Many of these older, urban hospitals, treating large percentages of Medicaid patients, provide relatively low-cost care. Renovating these hospitals would raise the costs of care; not renovating them would jeopardize patient care and safety; and closing them would leave large numbers of people with no other source of care. Other types of hospitals see new construction and modernization as tools in their marketing programs.

The concern with capital expenditure costs is based in large part on increases in operating costs which result from capital expenditure. Estimates of this increase vary, but it is composed of interest, depreciation, and the increased personnel and services required.

Another area of recent interest is the level of intensity and technology available in various types of institutions. Increasingly difficult medical feats can be carried out. Continued improvement in transplantation techniques and development of new and improved prostheses place more strain upon the financial resources of the system.

At the same time, new types of equipment provide more understanding of the physiological and biochemical processes. New technologies like Nuclear Magnetic Resonance (NMR) work to the advantage of organizations which are able to obtain them and to the disadvantage of smaller or poorer institutions which cannot. Institutions, through their administrators, need to work out reasonable arrangements for sharing new machines, skills, knowledge, personnel, and procedures. If they do not, new regulations will result because the primary payor, the federal government, has the power and will to control the costs resulting from introduction of new technology.

Competition has meant different things to those espousing it. Perhaps the best known proponent of competition in health care is Alain C. Enthoven, who has argued for allowing market forces to operate in the financing of health care services (4). Competitive pressures have entered health care as public policy and administrators are learning to become competitors.

Competition has increased at a number of levels. There is both inter- and intragroup competition among HMOs and HMO-like organizations and fee-for-service arrangements. The appeal of HMOs is not just cost. HMOs, particularly closed panel or staff ones, have considerable appeal to young and mobile Americans in terms of convenience, accessibility, and availability. Newcomers to an area are spared the necessity of locating a number of doctors and establishing contact with each. The single contact with an HMO, with some assurance of quality, is often crucual in the HMO decision.

The extent to which there is competition among different models of fee-for-service delivery varies across the country, but everywhere physicians are competing with more attractive office hours, and traditional emergency room patients are being attracted by Urgicenters or Emergicenters. Community and teaching hospitals are losing surgical patients with insurance to ambulatory surgical centers. Even the most traditional health care organizations are attempting to develop competitive strategies which will allow them to attract patients or clients and, where possible, patients or clients with insurance.

Acute-care hospitals, facing increased competition in their traditional services such as surgery and emergency care, increasingly seek to expand into other areas, with those which offer hope of profit being particularly attractive. With increased pressure on costs and constant attacks from competitors, hospitals seek to ensure a captive audience. One area with appeal is care for the elderly. Services supplied to the elderly might include institutional long-term care, home health services, congregate or other housing, meals and socialization activities (5).

A third level of competition lies in the structure and financing of health care. Enthoven has also addressed this area. Proponents of competition argue, legitimately, that the incentives have been misplaced, with providers passing costs on to insurers who pass them on to employers. Only very recently have employers, and employees, realized their role in this and taken steps to encourage a shift in incentives.

As part of the shifting of incentives, it has been suggested that consumers ought to be given a choice of levels of insurance with minimum catastrophic insurance, allowing consumers to choose the level of insurance they wish to purchase. Other suggestions include raising deductibles and coinsurance so as to give consumers larger stake in the decision to use care or not. Enthoven argues that the individual should be the customer for insurance, not the employer. This would shift some risk to consumers. While there is some interest in pursuing these issues, it is not clear what happens in cases where the individual is unable to pay after choosing a lower level of insurance. Nor is it clear whether increased control by insurers would result.

HMOs put providers at risk. Other types of organizations are being developed which will also put providers at risk. Preferred Provider Organizations are based on the premise that a low-cost health care organization or group of providers can benefit by delivering care to a group of people more cheaply in return for a monopoly on the provision of health care. The antitrust implications of such a monopoly have not been fully explored.

The next decade should see continued innovation in competitive practices and organizations. Providers in a more highly regulated, and at the same time more competitive, world will see whatever edge they can. That edge may be cost-based or service-based. As health care providers attempt to meet these challenges, they are likely to need different forms of organizations.

ORGANIZATIONAL CHANGES

There has been considerable discussion about multiinstitutional arrangements. The developments discussed above tend to encourage both horizontal and vertical integration.

Increasing numbers of hospital mergers are reported, and the aggregation of proprietary nursing homes has been rapid. In home health care there has been horizontal integration typified by merging Visiting Nurse Associations. This trend is likely to increase because larger organizations are probably more efficient as well as more powerful, and thus better able to withstand the pressures of cost control, regulation, and competition.

In the past there has not been much vertical integration, but this area is likely to show more growth in the future. If technology and highly specialized procedures are rationed, it seems likely that there will be a need for closer cooperation between the tertiary hospitals associated with medical schools and the community hosptials. Patient referral systems have not always worked well in the past, but payors may require such arrangements in the future, or financial incentives may make it worthwhile for the hospitals themselves to implement improved systems.

Hospitals will become more involved in long-term care in its broadest sense because they need to have an assured source of acutely ill patients and to move patients not acutely ill out of their beds as soon as possible. Hospitals are already involved with nursing homes, day care centers, home care, respite care, congregate housing, and housing for the elderly. Both proprietary and nonprofit hospitals would appear likely to benefit from such integration.

Health care providers also form a variety of other organizations for specific purposes. Buying cooperatives have existed for a number of years. Some hospitals share mobile CAT scanners. Some health care organizations sell services to others. Management services are already a common product offered and bought.

Corporate reorganizations are becoming common. These allow hospitals to benefit from associated activities which make a profit without jeopardizing their nonprofit status.

Health services administrators need to remain flexible and adaptable. Organizations need a strong sense of identity in order to decide what will or will not benefit them. Health care organizations, and their administrators, must resist becoming involved in activities which do not fit the organization. Administrators are required to assess their organization's major needs, and either join or develop organizational arrangements to meet them.

REFERENCES

1. Sager, "Urban Voluntary Hospitals."
2. Elpers and Crowell, "How Many Beds?"
3. Gibson and Walso, "National Health Expenditures," p. 2.
4. Enthoven, "Consumer Choice Health Plan" and "Consumer-Centered vs. Job-Centered Health Insurance."
5. Campion, Bang, and May, "Why Acute-Care Hospitals Must Undertake Long-Term Care."

Chapter 3

Health Services Administration

The activities of a health services administrator are usually classified in terms of function. Such classifications commonly begin with planning, proceed through variations of organizing, controlling, coordinating, leading, and end with evaluation.

The 1975 Commission on Education for Health Administration defined the process of Health Administration as "planning, organizing, directing, controlling, coordinating and evaluating the resources and procedures by which needs and demands for health and medical care and a healthful environment are fulfilled by the provision of specific services to individual clients, organizations, and communities" (1). The middle functions — organizing, directing, controlling, and coordinating — can be viewed as implementation or management.

PLANNING

Health services administrators have always planned. The planning process has been defined as: identification of the problem, gathering of data, development of alternative solutions, choice of alternative, and then evaluation. This traditional formulation did not include implementation, which was assumed. This process is similar to any problem-solving strategy, although the names given to each step and the number of steps vary from one author to another. Managers and administrators were taught to approach problems in this way, and it was often called planning. It was, however, an approach which centered on problems as they arose rather than on attempting to develop a strategy for controlling events.

Planning in health care has now taken on new meaning and has become a specialized activity, often carried out separately from other administrative functions. This institutional or strategic planning was derived from urban and comprehensive health planning initially, but has become more like the strategic planning done by leading business and industrial concerns.

The political and social philosophy of the United States was not compatible with the idea of social planning until well into the twentieth century. The beginnings of social planning lie in the urban planning begun in Chicago in the 1920s. The Depression and the Second World War delayed further progress while the anti-communism of the late forties and fifties prevented national planning, which was seen as an activity of communist or socialist countries.

Urban planning was revived in the 1950s, spurred partly by the problems resulting from the population migration to large northern cities. Housing received attention first, with substantial numbers of units of public housing built during this period, often as the result of large-scale plans.

In the 1960s there was a large increase in the areas in which national planning was done. Most of this effort was directed at urban areas with poor populations, with participation by those who were to be affected. Programs established poverty programs, urban redevelopment projects, pre-school education, and neighborhood health centers.

This trend toward national solutions for urban problems and the passage in 1965 of Medicare and Medicaid set the stage for passage of the Comprehensive Health Planning Act in 1966. The rationale for Comprehensive Health Planning (CHP) was that government was to pay a large share of the cost of health services, and, therefore, had an interest in seeing that the services provided were those which were appropriate to and needed by the community. The way to achieve this was seen to be the establishment of a board of local people who would monitor the system.

Comprehensive Health Planning was not a success. The resources and knowledge of individual CHP councils were far too small to enable them to even monitor, much less influence, the actions of large and powerful providers. Internal difficulties, partly the result of the way the legislation was written, allowed providers to dominate and operate the councils in their own interests.

CHP did highlight the need for people trained in health planning. Federal legislation provided some support for the training of health planners, and knowledge and expertise in the field began to develop. By the time the National Health Planning and Resources Development Act was passed in 1974, there appeared to be a sufficient base upon which to build an effective health planning system.

The law establishing Health Systems Agencies, P.L. 93-641, was vague and conflicting on the purposes of Health Systems Agencies (HSAs) and also on how they were to accomplish their objectives (2). It was definite about the structure of the agencies and about the professional staff which each agency was to have.

Each HSA was to have a minimum of five professional staff members, with an additional staff member for each 100,000 people in the health services area. As some HSAs had as many as 2,000,000 people in their areas, some staffs were as large as 20 or 25 professionals. Staff members were required to have expertise in health administration, the gathering and analysis of data, health planning, and the development and use of health resources (3).

By this provision health planning was closely tied to health administration, and many schools of health administration began specialty tracks in health planning. Courses in health planning became a required part of the curriculum for programs training health administrators.

The tie worked the other way as well. Health Systems Agencies provided state-of-the-art training and full-time experience to their staffs, many of whom later went to work for large health care provider organizations. Many of these former HSA staff members were hired initially to prepare Certificate of Need applications necessary to obtain approval for construction or changes in service.

This trend appears to have been very important in rapidly transporting the principles and methods of population-based planning from the HSAs to providers of health care. The comprehensive health planning done by health care providers rested on the same methodological and data bases.

Once poeple who identified themselves as planners were employed in health care organizations, they were open to the concepts of strategic planning.

Strategic planning involves defining the common mission or thread of the organization. According to Stoner, an organization which has identified its strategy correctly can survive tactical errors (4). A major purpose and consequence of strategic planning is explicit formulation of organizational goals and objectives. The process of formulation is itself helpful, but the setting of specific goals and objectives provides direction and purpose for the entire organization and a guide for evaluation. Strategic planning also defines how the organization proposes to meet its goals.

Strategic plans describe how the specific objectives are to be achieved. They list the resources — supplies, space, money, personnel — required. Strategic plans may include subobjectives which in sequence provide the timing or the phases of a project. For example, a goal aimed at stabilization of the financial status of a hospital might lead to an objective to increase occupancy in the pediatric unit by 5%. This might lead to a subobjective of recruiting two new pediatricians to the staff.

The implementation of a strategic plan which has well-developed objectives is less difficult than if objectives are not sufficiently defined. Because each objective contains its own built-in measure, evaluation consists of judging the extent to which the objective was achieved.

Both the setting of objectives and the implementation of a strategic plan will involve gathering of data and analysis of alternative choices. Administrators who become accustomed to thinking in terms of missions or purpose, goals, objectives, and strategies for meeting the objectives will also find it useful on a smaller scale. Strategic planning is an ongoing activity which takes place in a number of time frames and which is helpful in a variety of settings and situations. Administrators will find it useful to move the planning they do as part of their everyday routine closer to the model of strategic planning.

MANAGING

The task of management is ensuring that an organization performs effectively and efficiently (5). Attempts to describe management in functional terms — coordinating, controlling, organizing are not as helpful as they might be. They describe the purpose of the activity rather than the activity itself. The following discussion attempts to deal with the activities performed by the manager rather than the purpose. This seems a more useful classification to the authors for a number of reasons.

First, a description of the activities gives a better idea of what it is that a health services administrator does. It, therefore, provides the basis for the education which trains administrators. This enables the work of a health services administrator to be seen less as discrete areas, and more as the application of skills and knowledge to a variety of tasks and for a variety of purposes. It is useful to an administrator to be a good communicator, no matter what the purpose of the interaction.

The activities which make up management could be divided in a number of ways. As a first step in defining these activities, the authors have found it useful to use analysis, communication, facilitation and leadership, and decision making.

Analysis

Warner and Holloway provide a useful overview of analysis for decision making, dividing decisions into simple/complex and deterministic/stochastic. Thus, the number of variables and the randomness of the phenomena are accounted for. Warner and Holloway point out that,

> Most decisions that a health administrator or planner faces are stochastic and complex. It is, however, often desirable (because of costs) or mandatory (because of time and unavailable data) that the administrator *analyze* a complex stochastic decision as if it were simple and/or deterministic. Thus, our simple/complex, deterministic/stochastic characterization is applied to the *analysis* of the decision rather than to the decision itself (6).

The basic methods of quantitative analysis provide fairly clear-cut guidance for certain types of decisions. One such type is resource size decisions. These include different levels and mix of staffing, fixed cost/variable cost problems, scheduling, inventory, and problems involving minimizing resources or maximizing resources (7). It is these types of analyses which are used in the traditional function of control.

Excellent work has been done in applying some specific types of quantitative analysis to Health Services Administration. Warner and Luce have defined and examined the use of cost benefit and cost effectiveness analysis in health care. Dever has explored the role of epidemiological analysis in relation to community health, and work on the "new epidemiology" promises to lead to increased and better application of epidemiology (8).

An administrator may or may not do these analyses him/herself. An administrator needs to understand the components of these analyses and must have a role in determining their aims and objectives. The administrator must understand and in some cases will need to have a role in making assumptions which are used in the analysis. Administrators must also insist on sensitivity analysis for key variables. The implications of variable assumptions in financing, reimbursement, salaries, purchasing, and similar areas must be understood and examined. An administrator who depends on an analysis done by someone else and does not at least understand the major assumptions may end up making the wrong decision.

Analysis is less clear-cut when it addresses nonquantitative areas. The ultimate purpose of some analysts may be to quantify all variables, but few health services administrators will be ready to abandon nonquantifiable aspects of problems.

To an administrator making a decision on whether to start a new service or build a new building, a financial analysis giving projected surplus is only one of the factors to be considered. The administrator must survey the environment, consult with others who have a stake in the decision, and attempt an assessment of what others are doing — including actual or potential competitors or cooperators. He or she must study regulatory and governmental agencies and individuals and estimate potential changes. Organizations have often developed problems because they assumed a static environment or failed to estimate possible changes in the environment.

Consideration of these variables should include quantification whenever possible. An assessment of changes in the reimbursement system can be couched in probability terms. Similarly, the expectation that a competitor will enter a market can be put probabilistically. One can calculate the probability of events occurring which will lead to a favorable outcome, thus avoiding decisions based on a complex chain of events which is extremely unlikely to occur (9).

The role of the administrator is not primarily risk avoidance, but to encourage, demand, and perform realistic assessment of factors affecting future events. The role of the administrator is to assist in the assessment of variables where judgment and experience are required because quantified data is not available or is assumed.

An administrator who has observed a neighboring organization over the years, who knows the other administrator personally, and receives information from a variety of sources, explicit and implicit, can develop a subjective assessment of what the neighbor will do. If, however, the actions of the neighbor form a vital element in the decision, the administrator should be required to define his/her assessment probabilistically as well.

Communication

A large part of a health services administrator's time is spent communicating, verbally and in writing. It is likely that an administrator in the health care system spends a larger percentage of time in communication than do those who manage other types of organizations. The reasons for this include: the high percentage of work done by committees; the large number of internal and external constituencies which hold an administrator accountable; and the degree to which the delivery of health care remains a matter of interpersonal relations.

Administrators are more effective if they can speak and write well; inability to communicate may retard or end an administrator's career. Despite the importance of this aspect of an administrator's career, few educational programs deal adequately with it.

The emphasis within many educational programs is on writing papers of an academic nature. This is useful training for graduates: those going into policy analysis, for example, may find it necessary to be able to write a properly organized and documented academic paper. The practicing administrator, however, must also have the ability to write coherent and concise memos. This may often be as important.

The ability to communicate verbally, one-on-one or in groups, is extremely important to an administrator. Often an administrator will be called upon to make a formal presentation. At other times an administrator will want to persuade members of a group. In other situations an administrator may hold a discussion with an individual from whom the administrator hopes to gain information.

Students of Health Services Administration must practice these communication skills if they are to be good communicators. Students must have assignments where they write for a particular audience — an audience typical of the real world and not just that within the university. This is easy to do with cases, where the completion of the case might involve a memo to the administrator's superior or board. It is not necessary for faculty to see all the work that has gone into the analysis and conclusions; in most cases the student's work will be apparent. If calculations or similar parts of the work need to be shown, they can be put into an appendix to the case solution.

Students should be held to fairly regorous requirements on length — or rather on shortness. The most difficult thing for a student to learn may be what to leave out. The writing of long, well-researched and documented papers has its place, but so does the writing of short, precise pieces whose purpose is to convincingly present an analysis and recommend a course of action. In the latter, what is left out is important — not everything can be included. The ability to condense and combine where possible and to bridge the gaps left when information must be left out in the interest of brevity, comes with practice.

Students also need to practice appropriate types of oral communication. A form can be developed to evaluate students' oral presentations. If given to students at the time oral presentations are assigned, it will call their attention to important elements of the presentation, such as voice or appearance. When oral presentations are given, students should be held to strict time limits. Lengthy presentations tend not to be effective, and students can explore appropriate time limits for presentations of various types through a variety of assignments. A time limit which may seem too short to the speaker will often seem far too long to the listener.

Finally, students should receive practice in listening, in analyzing their own reactions to certain types of communications and to elements which affect them negatively and positively. Oral presentations in class can alert students to the way in which their personal characteristics and attitudes affect their reception of various types of communication. Practicing administrators also need to be alert to biases in their reception of communications so that they can be sure they are receiving the messages they need to be effective managers.

Facilitation and Leadership

A health services administrator is seen as one of the leaders of the organization and as such facilitates the work of others within the organization. The administrator is responsible for maintaining a broad perspective within the organization, emphasizing a proper balance between accountability to interests inside and outside of the organization and a primary sense of moral accountability.

The administrator relates to and works with organizations and individuals in the external environment whose functions or goals parallel or complement those of his/her own organization. The administrator aids and assists in the development of cooperative efforts, coordination of services, and sharing of services where appropriate.

To effectively fill the role of a facilitator, the administrator must encourage a process in which ideas can be expressed, different viewpoints examined, implications compared, consequences weighed, and ultimately solutions put forth. The goal of a facilitator is to encourage components within an organization or system to become more self-directed and to aid in developing and maintaining a flow of communication and cooperation that encourages and enhances effective and efficient performance and accountability.

Administrators cannot make every decision in an organization themselves. Development of personnel who are productive, satisfied, and able to make independent judgments when required is an essential part of the administrator's responsibilities. The health services administrator, as a facilitator, can add immeasurably to the development of a productive working environment that will encourage and assist personnel in striving toward professional effectiveness and responsibility.

Health services administrators are also responsible for facilitating change within their organizations. They must be able to stimulate change as well as set up an environment in which change is encouraged.

Organization development is an attempt to systematize change so that it does not have to be undertaken in crisis situations. It is not clear how successful health care organizations have been in setting up organization development efforts. Because of the number of actors whose agreement must be sought, the complexity of the structure of the health care system, and the extent to which the system is regulated, it is often a very slow process to initiate change in noncrisis situations. As a general rule, significant changes in health care organizations seems to take place when there is pressure from outside events rather than on a scheduled, ongoing basis.

It seems likely that as health care organizations set about redefining their missions and broadening their outlook and services, organization development will become more important, and those organizations which survive may well be those which are best able to plan for change within the organization.

In their role as leaders of the organization, administrators help set the tone for the organization. One of the major ways in which this is done is through selection, motivation, and evaluation of personnel. Selection and evaluation are sometimes handled by professional personnel administrators, although the ultimate responsibility is that of the Chief Executive Officer.

Selection involves recruitment, including a job analysis and job description, the actual recruitment from within or outside the organization, and the components of the selection process itself. This process may include: proficiency or other types of examinations, interviews, application form, reference and credential check, and the job offer. These are described in detail in Metzger's *Personnel Administration in Health Services Organizations* (35).

Evaluation of an employee's performance is important for a number of reasons. The evidence is that, if done properly, evaluation improves organizational effectiveness and individual employee performance (10).

Much material has been produced on the subject of motivation. Stoner defines motivation as ". . . that which causes, channels, and sustains people's behavior" and points out that old and new theories about what motivates employees ". . . differ in what they implicitly suggest managers should do to obtain effective performance from the people around them" (11). The theories differ in what they suggest managers should do because they differ in the assumptions they make about the motivation of employees. Veninga (48) has summarized these views and their implications for the health services administrator.

Decision Making

Decision making can be usefully divided into programmed and nonprogrammed decisions (12).

Programmed decisions are those which are made systematically in accordance with a set of rules. Modern organizations strive for the bureaucratic ideal where operations are governed by a consistent system of rules which are applied to specific cases. Such systematization brings with it equity, speed, and ease of decision making. Routines, policies, procedures, and sometimes custom or tradition contribute to these types of procedures.

Because programmed activity tends to drive out nonprogrammed activity, it is necessary that an organization and its administrators make special provision for the nonprogrammed decisions. Often this is expressed as the need for managers to set aside time to think, to plan, to read, and to engage in other activities which are preparation for important, nonprogrammed decisions.

Warner and Holloway (49) have discussed the types of quantifiable problems and analysis which lead to decisions in Health Services Administration. As their title, *Decision Making and Control for Health Administration*, implies, this type of decision making is intimately tied to control. These decisions tend to focus on delivery, scheduling, patient or product flow, revenues, expenditures, and other activities which can be easily quantified. Very sophisticated analytic models have been developed for measurement, forecasting, and control. Many of these systems involve feedback mechanisms which will automatically set into motion appropriate corrective actions.

Simon points out that every decision, even programmed ones, involves value elements (13). Factual elements lend themselves to quantification; value ones do not. Value elements, which include the goals of quantitative analysis, are less openly acknowledged, and the values may be those of organizations rather than individuals.

A community hospital faced with very high medical/surgical occupancy may choose any of a number of paths. Possible choices of action would include: building, attempts to reduce length of stay, merger or purchase of another facility, conversion of another service, or adoption of a closed staff model, to name only some. Although quantification of the effects of these alternatives can be done, the solution which is developed will have to be congruent with the values of that hospital if it is to be successful.

Some of the most important decisions which health services administrators make are nonprogrammed decisions, those which involve new types of policy decisions, one-chance opportunities, or cases in which it is not even clear whether or not a decision needs to be made. The necessity for making these types of decisions, particularly in the increasingly complex and changing world of health care, contributes to the view that administration is in large part an art. Traditionally, these decisions have been made largely on intuition and judgment or on the administrator's knowledge of similar situations.

Field placements of students in internships and residencies are to some extent designed to address these types of decisions. Students spend large amounts of time with their administrator preceptors because of the perceived necessity for future administrators to experience vicariously this type of decision making and to then begin making these decisions under the watchful eye of an experienced administrator.

Similarly, cases are used in the educational process to simulate nonprogrammed decisions. Cases usually devote considerable attention to the environment and political and organizational culture within which the case takes place because these are judged to be important elements in the solution of the case (14).

Although nonprogrammed decisions were in the past generally made in a nonsystematic way, this is changing. New analytical tools make it easier to consider options. Cost-benefit analysis, probabilities, computer simulations, and other linear programming techniques make it easier for the administrator to deal with some aspects of the one-time or nonprogrammed decisions.

EVALUATION

Evaluation is an essential competency for health services administrators. Evaluation involves "examining and weighing a phenomenon against some explicit or implicit yardstick" (15). Evaluation is also used to make choices among alternative courses of action.

Evaluation is similar to analysis except that evaluation includes an implication of decision making or action. "Evaluation as an applied research is committed to the principle of utility. It it is not going to have any effect on decisions, it is an exercise in futility" (16). Health services administrators who serve as Chief Executive Officers bear the delegated legal responsibility for the quality of care delivered by a health care organization. Quality assurance involves the measuring of services against established standards. Health services administrators also play major roles in the evaluation of personnel within an organization. In larger organizations the evaluation system may be established by personnel specialists; in smaller organizations the administrator will do it, perhaps with outside help. In either case, the administrator takes a lead role in evaluating those whom she/he supervises (17).

The evaluation of health programs for efficacy and efficiency is another important type of assessment (18). It is the final step in the process of program development and implementation. It is also a vital connection, feeding information back into planning and implementation activities.

Quantitative analysis done for the purposes of evaluation, as in choosing between alternative types of programs or measuring the cost-benefit ratio of a project or program, uses the same methods as analysis done for other purposes.

In health care organizations evaluation is also done as a basic requirement for certification and/or accreditation. Weiss points out other, covert reasons for doing evaluation, including: postponement, avoiding responsibility, public relations, and fulfilling grant requirements (19).

An essential element of evaluation is the standard against which things are measured. Evaluation usually measures process, organizational structure, or outcome. In some cases the standard will be prescribed, as with JCAH accreditation. In others, evaluation will be on how well the organization or program meets its own goals and objectives.

A different taxonomy of evaluation measures evaluation on its closeness to experimental research, or the degree of rigor. Thus, evaluation which is based on an experimental model is the purest; this is common in medical research, for example, new drug therapy. The closer the process is to experimental, the greater confidence we have that it is valid and unbiased (20). Within the health care system, however, many problems and processes will not be amenable to experimental design or to quasi-experimental design, even using simulation techniques. Some evaluation will always have to be done using case studies, anecdotal material, or subjective measures (21).

Evaluation is often discussed as if it were a discrete event, but it is an ongoing process measuring what is happening against what should happen, and then taking steps to restrict or reduce the discrepancies (22).

The amount of evaluation requiring an administrator's personal attention will vary from organization to organization and from administrator to administrator. Certainly, within each organization there needs to be continuous monitoring of revenue and expenditures in relation to the budget. Each organization may have its own particular trouble spot or spots, for example, patient census, physician productivity, ratio of Medicaid patients, nursing hours, number of ancillary services, or patient complaints. Once standards are established, procedures set up, and administrators satisfied that they or some other person within the organization will receive adequate notice of discrepancies, the system can operate with evaluation being integral and continual. However, there needs to be periodic evaluations of the adequacy of this system and adjustments made in what is being measured and how.

It is clear, then, that evaluation is not a magic formula which can only be carried out by experts or specialists in evaluation. It must be an integral part of what each administrator does.

REFERENCES

1. *Education for Health Administration*, p. 36.
2. Thompson, *Health Policy*, pp. 45-64.
3. P.L. 93-641, Section 1512 (b) (2).
4. Stoner, *Management*, p. 115.
5. Charns and Schaefer, *Health Care Organizations*, p. 225.
6. Warner and Holloway, *Decision Making and Control for Health Administration*, p. 48.
7. *Ibid.*
8. Crichton and Neuhauser, *The New Epidemiology*.
9. Pressman and Wildavsky, *Implementation*.
10. Veninga, *The Human Side of Health Administration*, p. 36.
11. Stoner, p. 405.
12. This is based on Simon, *The New Science of Management*, and Stoner.
13. Simon, *Administrative Behavior*, p. 45.
14. Hershey, *Hospital-Physician Relationships;* McConnell, *Health Care Supervisor's Casebook;* and Rakich, Longest, and Darr, *Cases in Health Services Management*.
15. Weiss, *Evaluation Research*, p. 1.
16. *Ibid.*, p. 10.
17. Metzger, *Personnel Administration in the Health Services Industry;* Veninga.
18. Borus, Buntz, and Tash, *Evaluating the Impact of Health Programs*.
19. Weiss, p. 10.
20. Campbell and Stanley, *Experimental and Quasi-Experimental Designs for Research*.
21. Borus, Buntz, and Tash, pp. 40-42; Weiss, pp. 73-78.
22. Hodgetts and Cascio, *Modern Health Care Administration*, pp. 296-297.

Chapter 4

Education

The Report of the Commission on Education for Health Services Administration, published in 1975, estimated that fewer than 25% of executive level positions in the health and medical care system were filled by individuals who possessed formal entry level education in health administration (1).

Health Services Administration is a profession that manages the system that delivers a broad range of health services to the public. The dynamic changes and increased demands that have occurred within the health care system, in the past decade alone, demonstrate that pressures are increasing for practitioners who have formal Health Services Administration education or who have updated their knowledge, skills, and attitudes.

Education for the health services administrator focuses on the fact that the main responsibility of the health services administrator is management (2).

> Management is not a static concept; it is rather a dynamic process which takes place in a social and political world. Management both creates and controls "change." With the ever-increasing rate of social and technological developments that are taking place in our time, management is THE central activity needed for human survival (3).

The effectiveness with which health services administrators manage and control health care organizations has tremendous implications. It is a vital factor in determining the survival of the organization and the quality of services it provides, and the ultimate survival of the health consumer, patient, or client.

To ensure effectiveness, practitioners must be trained and educated for their work roles. Society, and in particular those who pay for health care, expect professional health services administrators to possess effective management skills and competencies.

The educational foundation of Health Services Administration draws upon the knowledge and skills of several disciplines: economics, political science, medicine, engineering, epidemiology, organizational behavior, accounting, financial management, statistics, and computer technology. The relevant, well-planned educational program incorporates and integrates elements from each of these disciplines.

The health services administrator has a demanding and complex job which is carried out in a wide variety of continually changing settings. In order to be properly prepared to meet this challenge, the health services administrator needs educational preparation that is current, relevant, strong in the necessary basic foundation elements, and meets the needs of a dynamically changing health care system.

TYPES OF PROGRAMS

Baccalaureate Programs

Undergraduate degree programs in Health Services Administration have only been in existence since the early seventies. There has not been a large number of them so the number of graduates from these programs has been small. Therefore, it is not possible to assess their impact or draw valid conclusions about the positions ultimately to be held by bachelor degree holders.

A survey of the graduates of baccalaureate programs confirms the authors' experience that most graduates obtain entry- or mid-management level positions in health care facilities or organizations (4). Many of the respondents in the study had a sense of frustration that without a master's degree they were unable to obtain higher positions for which they felt adequately prepared.

The majority of undergraduate programs focus on the top management of less complex health care organizations and middle management of larger organizations. Perhaps the best opportunity for graduates with bachelor's degrees lies in the mid-management level opportunities within nursing homes, group medical practices, and unit management in hospitals. The unit management or department head responsibilities may be in central services, security, purchasing, admissions, or the business office.

Some undergraduate programs offer a bachelor's degree in Business Administration with a concentration in a more specific health-related area such as hospital accounting, health finance, or a similar field. The degree is basically a Bachelor's in Business Administration with a sequence of course work that is applicable to health organizations.

An undergraduate degree in Health Services Administration is not required as preparation for a graduate degree. There is not evidence that holding an undergraduate degree is a competitive advantage for admission into a graduate program. In fact, sometimes graduate programs prefer students from a broad-based, general education rather than from one designed for entrance on the bachelor's level. The articulation between undergraduate and graduate programs is an ongoing issue which the Association of University Programs in Health Administration and other professional bodies continue to address.

Health Services Administration programs can be situated in schools of Allied health, management, public health, public administration, or medicine. Program emphasis may reflect these locations. Students should seek programs which are consistent with their professional goals and philosophies.

A list of identified undergraduate programs can be found in Tourigny and LaFrance (47).

Graduate Programs

The master's degree in Health Services Administration is the most widely accepted professional preparation for a career managing health services. The number of Chief Executive Officers without such preparation is quickly being reduced, and graduate preparation in the field is being emphasized, encouraged, and often required.

Master's degree programs in Health Services Administration differ in content, title, and degree awarded. Examples of some degrees which are offered in the field are:

- Master of Health/Health Services Administration
- Master in Business Administration (in Health Administration
- Master of Public Administration
- Master of Science in Hospital/Hospital and Health Services/Health Care Administration
- Master in Hospital Administration
- Master of Arts in Health/Hospital/Hospital and Health Services/Health Care Administration
- Master of Public Health
- Master of Management in Hospital and Health Services Administration (5)

There is obviously a wide variety of options available. Desirable programs are those whose emphasis, objectives, and content permit flexibility and variety for the student with specific professional goals and background.

Accredited graduate programs, regardless of the degree awarded, require at least two years of full-time study or its equivalent. The programs include, in addition to the classroom academic requirements, a field practicum of varying length. The field practicum can be in the form of an administrative internship or an administrative residency.

The variety of available health administration programs allows students to choose a program that is of interest to them, builds on their previous educational experiences, and is in concert with their professional goals and objectives. This program variety and flexibility also ensures that the system has health administrative personnel with a diversity of approaches, talents, and perspectives.

In recent years there has been increasing interest in education at the doctoral level. Approximately ten universities have doctoral programs in Health Services Administration, and another twenty offer doctorates in related fields such as public health or business administration with emphasis on or specialization in health administration.

Graduates of doctoral programs are in demand as faculty members at universities and colleges, as researchers and consultants, and as practicing administrators. This level of education is likely to become more important as the field matures. A great deal of the research in Health Services Administration comes out of institutions with doctoral programs. In order for the field to gain credibility and recognition, emphasis on doctoral education and research must be emphasized and encouraged.

University faculty with doctorates in Health Services Administration rather than in foundation disciplines will do a great deal to produce practitioners with an integrated sense of the discipline. They will also encourage research that incorporates the knowledge from the contributing fields and builds on the conceptual framework of Health Services Administration.

Faculty trained in Health Services Administration will have a commitment to the discipline and a coherent sense of the future mission of the profession.

A list of member graduate programs can be obtained from the Association of University Programs in Health Administration (see Appendix I).

COMPETENCY-BASED EDUCATION

The recognition of limited resources in education has resulted in a great deal of emphasis being placed on the products or outcomes of the educational process. Competency- or performance-based instruction and/or education implies that the learning process results in a change in learner behavior. This suggests that, contrary to previously held expectations, the instructional process should have a tangible outcome (6).

Competency-based instruction is founded on educational theory developed by John Carroll and Benjamin Bloom. Effective instruction accommodates the learning style of individuals, with all their differences, in order that the majority of learners can master the competencies which the instructor wishes to convey. With this process, equal effort on the part of the instructor does not always result in equal student achievement (7).

Competency-based instruction is structured to offer uncomplicated availability to information and time to achieve mastery (8). This educational approach is directly related to the premise that all learning is based on specific objectives. When mastery of these objectives is demonstrated, the learner progresses to more complex objectives (9).

Competency-based instruction (CBI) is more a method than a program and has gained approval from accrediting bodies, legislators, and consumers of health care who are demanding accountability in programs that prepare health professionals. CBI is a step toward accomplishing this goal (10).

In education for Health Services Administration the desired objectives or outcomes tend to focus on the student's competencies in various aspects of planning, managing, and evaluating. Students may, for example, be asked to demonstrate their competency in decision making by doing a case. This might require them to use knowledge of organizational behavior, human resources management, health care finance, and health law to make a decision about a particular set of circumstances.

The desired competencies are developed on the basis of the expected activities of the health services administrator and, therefore, center on analysis, communication, leadership and facilitation, and decision making. The combination of skills, attitudes, aptitudes, and knowledge which comprise a competency are applied whether what is being done is planning, finance, personnel, or quality assurance.

PROGRAM FOUNDATIONS

The foundations of any educational program, regardless of the field, set the stage for all that is to follow. In order to develop a sound educational program in Health Services Administration, It is mandatory to address in sequential order: philosophy, program mission, goals, conceptual framework, and objectives. For examples of a philosophy and objectives see pages 70 and 71.

Philosophy

The primary step in designing an educational program is refinement and clarification of philosophical viewpoints (11). The institution and people developing the program address the issues relating to the philosophy of: society, education, the educational institution, and the school or college (if appropriate). From these underlying philosophical beliefs and statements evolves the philosophy of the program. Within this program philosophy the basic principles that are considered important to that program are articulated in a broad, general way. These principles reflect the values of the program as they relate to society and the maintenance and advancement of the social order. It answers the question: Why is the program important to society in general? What is its intrinsic value?

Mission Statement

The mission statement of the program evolves from the program philosophy. The mission statement establishes the main thrust and direction of the program in clear and concise language. It defines the prime purpose of the program and delineates its key functions or tasks.

Program Goals

The program goals evolve from the mission statement. These goals are stated in broad, general terms. They are the ideals for which the program will strive. These broad goals are guiding precepts for the development of the program and its curriculum. Frequently, goals and objectives are confused. Goals are broad-based ideals that give general direction to a program. All of the program goals may not be attained. This does not mean that the program is not sound or effective.

Conceptual Framework

The logical progression from the program philosophy, mission statement, and program goals is the development of the conceptual framework of the program. This framework focuses on broad content areas or disciplines that will be addressed within the total program including the basic ideas or concepts that contribute to the total program. The development of a framework is necessary and based on the premise that the concepts addressed are meaningful and significant elements contributing to the educational soundness of the program.

The conceptual framework enumerates all of the broad educational disciplines that will be drawn upon to contribute the basic theory to the overall program content. This would include, but not be restricted to, the specialty area or areas. All contributing educational fields would be clearly defined in this statement.

Incorporated within the conceptual framework is the identification of the major concepts of the program. These main ideas or basic theory threads are the key building blocks upon which the entire program is structured.

After the major concepts are articulated, the curriculum strands of the program must be identified and developed. These strands are either horizontal or vertical in nature. The horizontal curriculum strand or strands are the key elements that are given equal emphasis in every major course. An illustration of a horizontal strand could be the Health Services Administration process.

The vertical strand or strands are initially taught in introductory courses as basic concepts with additional, more complex content introduced during each of the subsequent professional courses in a progressive and sequential manner. There are usually more vertical than horizontal strands. Vertical strands could include evaluation or management (12).

Objectives

Bloom's *Taxonomy of Educational Objectives* provides the foundation for any discussion of educational objectives (13). Bloom directed educators to focus instructional objectives on the competencies exhibited by learner outcomes instead of the presented content. All educational objectives can be developed in terms of measurable behaviors, and all learning is classified in one of three domains: cognitive, affective, or psychomotor.

"The *cognitive domain* includes those objectives which deal with recall or recognition of knowledge and the development of intellectual abilities and skills" (14). Most Health Services Administration education is within the cognitive domain.

The cognitive taxonomy is arranged in six major classes which move from the simple to the complex, from the concrete to the abstract. They range from knowledge which involves the recall of specific factual information to evaluation which involves quantitative or qualitative judgments (15).

The affective domain includes those objectives which emphasize values, interests, attitudes, emotions, or feelings (16).

They psychomotor domain includes those objectives which emphasize some muscular or motor skill, some manipulation of materials and objects, or some act which requires neuromuscular coordination (17).

Behavioral objectives contain content and an expected behavioral change in the learner due to change in knowledge, attitudes, values, or skills (18). Behavioral objectives have a good deal of flexibility, and they can be as broad or as specific as the educator needs or desires. They can also be tailored to the appropriate learner: student, client, adult, employee, or patient. In Health Services Administration educational objectives represent the competencies desired for students completing the program.

One of the keys to writing and developing good behavioral objectives is to select the proper verbs, those which describe cognitive processes (19). The verb which is used in writing a behavioral objective needs to be clearly measurable. The verb that is used in the behavioral objective spells out the manner in which evaluation of that objective takes place, for example: to describe, to analyze, to illustrate, to list (10). Behavioral objectives can be developed for a program, a unit, a lesson, or other element of the educational process.

Some educators do not agree that behavioral objectives are necessary or even desirable in the educational process. The authors believe that sound educational instruction clearly informs the learner what will be achieved and how it will be achieved. Behavioral objectives also assist the educator to structure the learning experiences, give guidance to the necessary content to be included, and provide clear direction as to the method of evaluation. Behavioral objectives streamline the instructional process, clarifying the purpose and intent of learning for the educator and student, and make both accountable for achieving desired ends.

EDUCATIONAL EVALUATION

Evaluation in education is a process of juding the effectiveness of the educational experience (21) and involves more than just the mechanics of testing.

Evaluation assists in identifying positive and negative areas (22). For too long and too often evaluation has been focused on the negative. The positive must and can be acknowledged.

There are five important principles that are particularly important in evaluation of education where the desired outcomes are increases in competency:

1. Evaluation is continuous and concurrent.
2. Evaluation is concerned with outcomes, structure, and process.
3. Evaluation is cooperative. All who are affected by the evaluation should participate.
4. Evaluation focuses on important values. These are often stated as goals or objectives (23).
5. Evaluation is formative (during) and summative (completion).

Evaluation is a cyclical, ongoing process. Evaluation is maintained throughout the educational experience. At times it may be desirable and appropriate to have a pre-evaluation or post- or post-post-evaluation as well as formative and summative evaluations. Examples of evaluation instruments are given on pages 99-103 and 105-106.

Evaluation procedures are imperfect and should be placed in the proper context. They can provide necessary and valuable information, but they should not be regarded as final and ideal. Evaluation, in any context, needs to be based on specific objectives. Without this, evaluation becomes purposeless, or the end rather than the means to that end. It is a tool of assessment which adds a measure of appraisal, clarity, and validity to any endeavor.

CONTINUING EDUCATION

The health services administrator has a responsibility to continue his or her education. As a member of a profession which has developed rapidly in the past twenty hears, the health services administrator already in the field needs to participate in activities which will keep his or her knowledge current.

Because the field of Health Services Administration is new and developing rapidly, members of the profession can expect major developments in theory, research, and practice within the coming years. Administrators have to undertake continuing efforts to stay abreast of these developments. One of the most important ways is through continuing education which can provide new information and skills in a relatively short period of time.

Health services administrators need continuing education to stay abreast of developments which impinge upon their administrative tasks, but which may not be of primary importance to them. Such areas, varying from administrator to administrator and from organization to organization, may include, for example, technology assessment, planning and marketing, quality assurance, or reimbursement.

New knowledge and skill can be gained from seminars, short courses, workshops, conferences, or by attendance at other activities sponsored by professional societies, government bodies, or universities. The administrator should apply to these activities the same evaluation criteria used in selecting more formal education. Objectives need to be clearly stated, those teaching should be qualified, there should be some form of evaluation, and there should be opportunities for the participants to apply what they have learned, particularly if skills are involved.

At some point in their professional lives administrators may find it useful or necessary to make a more sustained educational commitment and seek another degree or participate in a more extensive, specialized program. By doing this the administrator will be able to develop a new theoretical and conceptual framework, replacing what is out of date. Such a framework will assist the administrator in his dealings with complex organizations in changing environments.

For example, an administrator trained before the development of comprehensive health planning may not be able to deal with planning issues as effectively as the administrator with a better grounding in the field. A more comprehensive approach would provide the administrator with the historical perspective to place strategic planning within a developmental context, and enables him/her to incorporate relevant elements from strategic planning to his/her own organization and to deal better with regulatory and planning agencies.

Administrators also need to be aware of the special continuing education requirements connected with their fields of specialization. Licensed nursing home administrators are usually required to obtain continuing education credits, and membership in some professional organizations depends on this participation.

Some organizations will provide financial incentives for administrators to continue their education. Tuition is often paid, and salaries, benefits, or promotion may well be tied to educational accomplishments as well as to performance.

Administrators also have a responsibility for ensuring the continuing education of their organization's staff. In–service education needs to be a regular part of most health care organizations.

The working out of such arrangements is seldom the direct responsibility of the health services administrator, but she/he is one of those who set the tone for the entire organization. This is best accomplished by support of continuing education and by setting an example through the administrator's own continuing education efforts.

Practicing health services administrators also have an obligation to assist in the development of their profession. Because Health Services Administration is eclectic, drawing from other fields, and because of its recent origins, it is not as fully developed as other professions. There are particular weaknesses in theory and research.

Health Services Administration is based largely on the theory of other disciplines. Perusal of the major texts in Health Administration shows, for example, considerable reliance on the application of organizational theory to health care organizations and some consideration of the concerns of medical sociologists, with no real integration. A great deal of theoretical work remains to be done to make this as useful as possible to administrators.

Similarly, Health Services Research is relatively underdeveloped, and the bulk of research carried out on the administration of health services has emanated from those in other disciplines — medicine, management, economics, operations research, or sociology, for example — and has, therefore, lacked the integrating capacity which is one of the hallmarks of Health Services Administration.

As doctoral programs in Health Services Administration expand, it is expected that faculty and students in those schools, as well as in those schools preparing students at the master's level, will devote more attention to both theory and research. As these developments take place, the health services administrator in the field needs to undertake continuous efforts to evaluate the relevance of this work and to provide assistance to theoreticians and researchers. Practicing health services administrators are likely to feel less comfortable and demonstrate less interest in these responsibilities than those requiring upgrading of financial or management skills. All aspects — practice, theory, and research — are necessary for a viable, current, and dynamic professional discipline.

ACCREDITATION

The Accrediting Commission on Education for Health Services Administration (ACEHSA) controls accreditation of educational programs in health administration. Only graduate programs are eligible for accreditation, and they are not eligible until at least one class has graduated.

Accreditation is based on an intensive survey questionnaire and an on-site visit by representatives of ACEHSA. Site visits are usually made by a team of three members: a member of the Commission, a director or senior faculty member of an accredited graduate program, and the Executive Secretary of the Commission or his representative.

The members of the site-visit team apply the criteria to the objectives, mission, and purposes of each program, and attempt to provide sufficient flexibility within the criteria to allow for differences in setting and resources and to encourage innovation in education for Health Services Administration.

Following the site visit, a report is prepared by the Commission and sent to the program for review. The program responds to the report, presenting plans to follow up on specific suggestions made by the Commission. Each program is required to submit a progress report to the Commission one year after receipt of the Commission's report.

This approach by the Commission is designed to stress self-evaluation and ". . . to greatly strengthen a Graduate Program and further its goals" (24).

The accreditation criteria address resources of the university and program; accreditation status of the university and specialized college; the curriculum of the program; the faculty and its participation in research, community service, and continuing education; criteria and procedures for selection, retention, and evaluation of students; and program evaluation. Accreditation may be for a period of up to seven years.

The Accrediting Commission is directed by a Board which includes representatives of its member organizations and two public members. Each member organization is entitled to one seat on the Board, except for the Association of University Programs in Health Administration (AUPHA), which has four seats and votes. Founding members of the Commission were AUPHA, the American College of Hospital Administrators, the American Hospital Association, and the American Public Health Association. Organizations which have joined since then include the American Health Planning Association, the American College of Nursing Home Administrators, the Association of Mental Health Administrators, and the American College of Medical Group Administrators.

Staff for the ACEHSA is supplied by the Association of University Programs in Health Administration, and the two organizations have offices together. The Commission has three Fellows each year who do much of the work of the Commission. These are often young faculty members from members of AUPHA.

The Accrediting Commission is supported by dues from member organizations, fees for evaluation site visits, and by other income.

THE ASSOCIATION OF UNIVERSITY PROGRAMS IN HEALTH ADMINISTRATION (AUPHA)

The Association of University Programs in Health Administration (AUPHA) is the umbrella organization for programs educating health administrators.

AUPHA was formed to promote improvement in graduate, baccalaureate, and continuing education programs in health administration, to aid the development of the discipline, and to increase recognition of the importance of professional administration in health.

AUPHA has been instrumental in the development of the profession, plays a central role in the accreditation of programs in Health Services Administration, and speaks and acts for those concerned with education in the field.

Activities

The organization views itself as having a number of major functions, the emphasis on these varying with the resources available and the perceived need. Although AUPHA seeks to act in concert with other organizations, it is the only organization which speaks for the whole field of Health Services Administration.

AUPHA's primary purpose is improvement of education in Health Services Administration. It also helps to make education for Health Services Administration more accessible; it has done considerable work to encourage qualified people to pursue education in Health Services Administration.

A major portion of the activities of the organization have centered on curriculum development. A number of task forces have been organized and have made contributions in defining curriculum content. The Task Force on Financial Management Education, one of the most recent, produced a book (54) which is extremely helpful to those planning or teaching courses in the subject. Other task forces have focused on Home Health Agency Administration, Mental Health/Mental Retardation Administration, and Long-Term Care, to name just a few.

Conferences, committees, and seminars have dealt with other subjects of importance to Health Services Administration and have provided information and stimulus to those involved in education for the field. Subjects have included Health Law, Health Policy, Non-Traditional Education, Undergraduate Education, Research Policy, and Quality Assurance.

Institutes sponsored by AUPHA have provided faculty members with new skills and knowledge and often bring together educators and practitioners. Institutes have centered on Financial Management, Case Method Teaching, the Use of Microcomputers, and similar topics.

The second major function of AUPHA is dissemination of new knowledge in the field. AUPHA accomplishes this through institutes, seminars, presentations at the annual meeting, and by its publications. AUPHA publishes a number of books, a listing of member programs throughout the world, and promotional literature aimed at recruitment of students. AUPHA publishes the *Journal of Health Administration Education* and plans to move more aggressively into journal publication in the future.

AUPHA also co-sponsors, with the Bureau of Hospital Administration at the University of Michigan, the Health Administration Press, founded in 1972 and located in Ann Arbor. The Press, partly funded by the Kellogg Foundation, publishes books on health administration, many of them basic texts used in health administration courses. The Press also publishes three journals: *Health Care Research*, *Medical Care Research*, and *Abstracts of Health Care Management.*

AUPHA also acts as a central resource and represents programs providing education for Health Services Administration. This includes lobbying, particularly for increased or sustained funding, encouraging exchanges of knowledge among programs, and attempting to educate those outside the field about the importance of quality professional education in health administration.

AUPHA plays a dominant role in the Accrediting Commission on Education for Health Services Administration (ACEHSA). As discussed previously, four members of the Commission represent AUPHA, and a member of the AUPHA staff is Executive Secretary of the Commission. The offices of the two organizations are located together.

While the symbiotic relationship between the two organizatins may be necessary and is certainly convenient, it presents some potential dangers that the affairs of the two organizations will not be kept separate and that events and circumstances within AUPHA will influence the accreditation process.

AUPHA defines part of its mission as anticipating future needs and promoting strategies to meet them. Many of the activities already discussed fulfill these aims, but efforts by the Association to achieve firm financial support for Health Services Administration education should be noted particularly.

The Association collects data on a number of issues. Frequent surveys are done of graduate job placements, and in 1983 a survey of baccalaureate program graduates was published (47) (25). Faculty salary surveys are done, and a yearly survey collects and distributes data from each program on such issues as faculty and student numbers and financial support for the program.

Finally, AUPHA is dedicated to promoting Health Services Administration education on an international basis. Under contract from the Agency for International Development (AID), a number of conferences, workshops, and other activities have been carried on outside of the United States, but such activities have been curtailed because of lack of funding. However, there are international members of AUPHA, and the Association is clearly committed to supporting and assisting those working in the field abroad.

Organization

There are a number of membership categoreis in AUPHA. Although individual memberships are available and some organizations such as state hospital associations are also members, most membership is by educational program. Type A members are fully accredited graduate programs. Type B are approved undergraduate programs. There is no accreditation for undergraduate programs, but Type B members must meet a set of requirements established by AUPHA. These are considerably less rigorous than standards for graduate accreditation and do not include a site visit, although the need for a site visit has been discussed within AUPHA.

Type C memberships, both graduate and undergraduate programs, include those who do not meet the requirements for Type A or Type B membership. This category allows programs to receive the benefits of AUPHA membership while they are attempting to meet the requirements. In fact, it would be difficult for a program to meet the requirements if it did not have such access. However, programs may not remain indefinitely as Type C members. If fairly rapid progress is not made out of Type C membership, programs' membership is terminated.

There are also international memberships and memberships for programs which do not grant degrees in Health Services Administration.

There are some problems with this structure. First, because membership in AUPHA is relatively expensive, there is a resulting bias within the organization toward the older, more established, wealthier graduate programs. The second problem is that by requiring programs to become Type A or Type B members fairly rapidly or be excluded, AUPHA is maintaining standards, but leaving some programs without help which they badly need. It may be in the very programs which cannot or will not meet accreditation or membership standards that most need the help AUPHA can offer. If AUPHA hopes to raise standards of education for Health Services Administration, it needs to address the whole spectrum of educational programs, not just those able to meet its standards easily or quickly.

There does appear to be increased emphasis within AUPHA on baccalaureate education and more talk of the need for qualified health services administrators throughout the whole range of the health care system, not just in hospitals. The latter does not appear to have permeated the organization, as a perusal of topics discussed at annual meetings, seminars, and other gatherings will indicate. Striking the balance will be difficult as attempts to contain costs will continue to focus attention on acute–care hospitals, thus reinforcing the existing bias of the organization.

AUPHA has a eight–person Board of Directors. The Chairperson, Past Chairperson, Chairperson Elect, President, and four members elected by the membership at large are members. At least one of the members of the Board must come from an undergraduate program. Only full–time faculty of member programs may serve on the Board.

The affairs of the Association are managed by a President and Vice President. In addition to the Office of the President and a Resource Center, there are special offices for Management, Undergraduate Education, Research and Student Affairs, Educational Opportunity, and Financial Management Education.

The work of the Association is funded in part by members' dues and in part by outside income. Some of this is obtained in the form of contracts, but much is contributed. In the past, the Association received large sums from the Kellogg Foundation, but the termination of that support has resulted in the need to raise money from the corporate sector. Because of the increasing interest in cost containment and the obvious connection that the business community can make between cost containment and good management, the Association has been reasonably successful in obtaining this support.

The need for the Association will continue, but is will face difficult challenges. Increasing competition for the declining school–age population threatens to pit program against program. Decreasing federal and state government aid for higher education threatens some of the larger, more extablished programs which have contributed greatly to the Association in the past.

AUPHA is faced with attempting to promote and maintain quality standards of education for Health Services Administration at a time when an increasing number of students and programs will be seeking innovative ways to respond to a rapidly changing environment. Balances will be hard to strike, but the Association must do so if it is to continue its important role in the development of the discipline.

REFERENCES

1. *Education for Health Administration*, p. 6.
2. Levey and Loomba, p. 491.
3. *Ibid.*, pp. 491-492.
4. Tourigny and LaFrance, *Baccalaureate Health Administration Graduates.*
5. Bellin and Weeks, pp. 3-4.
6. Ford and Morgan, *Teaching in the Health Professions*, p. 2.
7. *Ibid.*
8. *Ibid.*, p. 3.
9. *Ibid.*, p. 34.
10. *Ibid.*
11. Willgoose, *Health Teaching in Secondary Schools*, p. 61.
12. University of Lowell, Master's of Science in Health Services Administration.
13. Bloom, *Taxonomy of Educational Objectives.*
14. Bloom, *et al.*, *Taxonomy*, *Handbook 1*, p. 7.
15. *Ibid.*, pp. 62, 185.
16. Krathwohl, *et al.*, *Taxonomy Handbook 2*, p. 116.
17. *Ibid.*, p. 7.
18. Willgoose, p. 45.
19. *Ibid.*, p. 52.
20. For a list of verbs to be used in writing behavioral objectives, see Scott and Carlo, *On Becoming a Health Educator*, p. 55.
21. Willgoose, p. 380.
22. Bruess, *Implementing Comprehensive School Health*, p. 338.
23. *Ibid.*
24. Accrediting Commission on Education for Health Services Administration, "The Accreditation Process."
25. Tourigny and LaFrance.

Chapter 5

Field Placements: Internships and Residencies

A field placement has been a part of education for health administrators for many years. It generally has been required because administration was seen as an art as well as a science. The need to integrate material from a variety of disciplines into the practice of health administration has added to the perceived need for an apprentice period.

The persistence of field placements in the training of health services administrators is an indication that field placements fulfill the needs of those involved in such experiences. For those in the field already, the field placement, residency, or internship at least in part represents an initiation rite. This is a common denominator for those who enter the field, as well as a bond.

For those who act as preceptors, the supervisors in the field experience, the experience offers a number of advantages. Many preceptors enjoy teaching; others may gain from the connection with a university or college. The rewards may include adjunct or other faculty status, intellectual stimulation, and the opportunity to teach or lecture within the program. Many administrators feel that having a student stimulates them to question their actions and performance and generally improves their organization.

Preceptors may also use the field experience as a screening for future employment, either for their own organization or for organizations in which they have colleagues. A promising resident or intern may be hired by the organization in which the field work is done, but it is more common for a preceptor to recommend a promising student to someone who is known to have a vacancy.

Programs in health administration gain from their system of field placements, and progams are judged partly on the basis of the organizations in which their students are placed. Supervision of field placements, particularly the closer supervision required in undergraduate programs, results in an interchange between faculty and administrators which improves education for administration.

Programs training administrators as well as program faculty gain in a number of ways from this apprentice system. It enables them to pass on to practicing administrators partial responsibility for the practical aspects of the education of their students. More importantly, faculty develop a network of providers who are then available to act as guest lecturers or speakers, to employ graduates of the program, to assist or facilitate research by faculty and students, and to act as a friend of the program should it be threatened. Programs facing decreasing revenue from federal and state governments and declining student enrollments are likely to find the latter important.

Students in the field placement also gain, although in the longer residencies students may find that the benefits are outweighed by the costs. Through the field placement, students gain experience which is very close to that which they would obtain in a job. For those who have not previously worked in an administrative position, the field work may be accepted as a substitute for needed experience. Students have an opportunity to develop skills and interests and to integrate the academic training they have received.

In addition, students are given a look at a health care organization from a much greater height within the organization than the level at which they would enter as employees. This knowledge of what goes on at higher levels of administration will enable the new administrator to perform better. The preceptor may act as a mentor for the student, even after the internship ends, and many students continue to seek advice and support from the preceptors on difficulties encountered as well as on the future course of their careers.

Many preceptors also help those who have done placements under them to obtain jobs. They provide recommendations, contacts, and introductions.

Finally, the field placement provides students with the opportunity to observe and learn from what may be viewed as a master administrator. The student also has the opportunity to try out different styles him/herself, to try various approaches and ways of solving problems and making decisions, and to observe the effect and outcome.

The origins of Health Service Administration field placements were in the one- or two-year residencies done by those trained as hospital administrators. In these residencies, students were assigned to an administrator who supervised their residency. While some of the time in the residency was spent with the administrator (for example, attending staff meetings) and some of the time in the completion of a specific project, a great deal of time was spent in rotating through the hospital. The purpose of the rotation was to ensure that the future hospital administrator, presumably a future Chief Executive Officer (CEO), knew what went on in every part of the hospital.

With this in mind, residents traditionally spent a specified period in the laundry, in the dietary department, with the nursing staff, and so on. As hospitals have become more complex and the number of departments has grown, this has obviously resulted in less time spent in more departments.

This model of the residency has persisted for some time in acute-care hospitals and nursing homes. Preceptors often copy their own residency experience without thinking about whether it is really necessary for a Chief Executive Officer to know all about the dietary department, or whether, in fact, the student in the residency will ever become a CEO.

As training specifically for administration of health care services other than hospitals has developed, the field experience has become more flexible. Students training to be nursing home administrators are normally required to do an internship of six months, although various states have different requirements for those enrolled in accredited educational programs. It is also possible in some states to become a nursing home administrator by completion of an internship which is not connected to an educational institution (1).

Residency or internship requirements for those training as administrators of medical groups, HMOs, health centers, mental health facilities, or clinics are not set; this gives faculty, students, and preceptors considerable latitude, but probably requires more careful supervision of the experience than has been usual in residencies in hospitals.

COMPARISONS OF INTERNSHIPS AND RESIDENCIES

Internships and residencies differ largely on the length of the experience and remuneration received. Residencies generally last at least one year and sometimes two, are full-time, and the student resident is remunerated. Internships last for varying periods of time, may be part-time or full-time, and may or may not involve payment to the intern. While residencies are usually done after the completion of all course work, internships often are done concurrently with course work.

As programs training health services administrators become more varied (an example being external degree programs) and an increasing number of programs are aimed at the person already working in the field, scheduling difficulties may result in shorter internships or residencies, or the substitution of other requirements in place of a field practicum. As programs train students for jobs in a variety of settings other than acute-care hospitals, residencies and internships may hold a different value than they have in the past.

At the present time a field experience is not required for accreditation of graduate programs in Health Services Administration, although it is considered desirable. Undergraduate programs wishing to become full members of AIPHA (see page 45) must include a field experience in their curriculum.

THE ROLE OF THE STUDENT, FACULTY, AND PRECEPTOR

In an internship or residency, faculty, students, and preceptors have mutual obligations. The responsibility for specific tasks may vary among types of organizations and the nature of the field practicum. See pages 89–92 for one listing of these.

Generally, in a residency there will be less supervision by the program faculty once the student is in the placement while undergraduate internships will be closely supervised by program faculty. Therefore, internships are generally done within close distance of the college of university, while residencies may be done in facilities or agencies which are far afield.

The Responsibility of Program Faculty in the Field Experience

Placement. The first responsibility of the faculty is to provide a field placement for each student. In some programs students may be asked to find their own placement with program approval. Faculty must be prepared to place those students who are not able to locate an internship or residency placement on their own.

Faculty are also responsible for ensuring the quality of the placement. There are several components. There must be some assurance that the preceptor is qualified. Generally, preceptors will be asked to supply a resume or curriculum vita giving their qualifications. At a minimum the preceptor should be trained to the level of the program. That is, a student completing a master's program should not be assigned to a preceptor who does not have at least a master's degree. The reason is that graduate training emphasizes different areas and more specialization than does undergraduate training. An exception might be made for exceptional preceptors, but these should be based on the characteristics of the preceptor, not the convenience of the students or the program.

Additionally, the program faculty must assure that the organization to which the student is being sent is of satisfactory standing. At a minimum, facilities or agencies should be accredited or certified as necessary. Faculty will have to use their own judgment to establish other criteria, which should include the likelihood that the student will have a positive educational experience.

It might be assumed that organizational stability would be a requirement. This need not be the case, however. While students should not be sent to organizations which appear to be in great disorder, some students may benefit from placement in a challenging situation. In organizations undergoing great change, the student has the opportunity to observe what happens in situations which are becoming less rare, e.g., change in Chief Executive Officer or receivership in a nursing home, and may also be given more interesting work to do because of the situation. Program faculty will need to keep closely in touch with placements where such situations occur and decide what to do on the basis of their knowledge of the situation and the student and in conjunction with placement personnel.

The program should provide a Memorandum of Agreement or a contract to be signed between the organization in which the student is placed and the educational institution and program. Program faculty may wish to arrange for liability insurance to cover students and themselves.

Program faculty assume the responsibility for ensuring that students who are not adequately prepared are not placed in internships. This means that program faculty must adopt a standard for retaining students in the program and must grade in courses so as to eliminate those students who are not capable of becoming health services administrators.

Faculty must supervise the internships to the extent necessary to ensure that the internship progresses satisfactorily and that difficulties or conflicts that may arise are resolved in a positive manner.

Program faculty or staff are responsible for carrying out the administrative work associated with the placement and its requirements, providing evaluation forms and schedules, and arranging for the preceptor to receive whatever measure of thanks or reward is provided. This may include adjunct faculty status, course vouchers, or contributions to the organization.

Faculty need to be prepared to make necessary periodic changes in placement sites. As individuals and organizations change, placements may need to be eliminated or replaced by new or better ones. Faculty will wish to keep some balance among types of organizations. This is particularly helpful where seminars are run concurrently with the field placements. Organizations such as HMOs, hospices, urgent care or walk-in centers, and medical group practices, which are becoming more important, need to be represented in the program placements, and programs may also wish to focus on less traditional areas such as home health or community-based mental health agencies.

Supervision. Undergraduates are supervised more closely in their field placements than are graduates. Some elements of supervision pertain to all field experiences.

For every internship or residency there should be a series of reports to program faculty outlining what is being done in the placement. Undergraduate programs usually include a more detailed report than do graduate programs. If there are enough faculty, it may be helpful to have undergraduate students keep journals rather than logs. This encourages a dialogue between students and faculty and allows faculty to channel students' thinking so that better integration between the academic work and the field is achieved. The practice in writing, if corrected by faculty members may be better able to pinpoint students who need remedial work in writing and organization.

In the case of undergraduates particularly, attention needs to be given to the emotional responses of students exposed personally for the first time to issues surrounding serious illness or death. Those students who are in nursing homes or hospices will need special monitoring. Faculty and preceptors both need to be alert to potential problems in this area; a journal permits faculty to have a better idea of the thinking of students.

In addition to periodic reporting on the field placement, it is helpful if students and faculty meet regularly. This is more usual with undergraduate programs than with graduate ones, where students are sometimes placed at great distances. Periodic seminars allow students to compare experiences and generalize from a larger sample.

Program faculty may play a major role where field placements are not going well. Adequate supervision allows faculty to identify internships or residencies that are in difficulty early. Usually a faculty member is able to intervene successfully, although sometimes a student may have to change placements. Field placements most often have trouble because of personality conflicts between preceptor and student, the student's inability to deal with issues within the placement setting (for example, in a hospice), or differing expectations between student and preceptor. Program faculty can most successfully intervene in the latter case. Experience in supervision on the part of faculty will improve their ability to match students with preceptors and placements, and also allow them to spot difficulties early and to act successfully to improve the situation.

The faculty may also wish to make assignments which will heighten the field experience for the students. Well-designed problems, cases, or paper assignments may encourage students to better analyze and understand the organization in which they are placed. Such assignments should encourage students to critically examine what is happening around them. For examples see pages 95-96 and 97-98.

Evaluation. Faculty need to develop and oversee periodic evaluation of the field placement.

Students in the field placement should be evaluated on criteria which are related to and drawn from the projected outcomes or program objectives for students. The evaluation forms should be distributed to preceptors and students at the beginning of the field placement to ensure that both parties know the criteria on which evaluation is based. For an example see pages 99-103.

Students should also be asked to evaluate their placement and preceptor. This evaluation is helpful to program faculty in making future placements and in placing the preceptor's evaluation of the student in context, and it contributes to total program evaluation.

The Responsibility of the Preceptor in the Field Experience

Health services administrators, like members of other professions, have an obligation, and ideally a desire, to assist in the training of new members of the profession. This will often be done by serving as a preceptor for internships or residencies done by students in Health Services Administration.

The requirement for internships or residencies recognizes that successful administration requires practice, not just academic knowledge. It also recognizes that this practice is best provided under the direction of an experienced administrator. There is no substitute for this practical experience.

Many administrators find that acting as a preceptor stimulates not only them, but others in their organization. Most administrators who act as preceptors are good teachers and enjoy the challenge of explaining to a student practices they may have taken for granted. Such administrators feel that the rewards of preceptorship far outweight the heavy responsibility it entails.

In accepting an intern or student, the preceptor accepts the day-to-day responsibility for the student. This involves concern for the emotional well-being of the student in addition to his/her professional and intellectual development.

The primary task of the preceptor is to supervise the growth and development of the student. In some areas the preceptor will want to teach in a didactic or Socratic way, in others, to arrange for the intern or resident to learn by doing. The preceptor will want to establish some checkpoints against which to measure the student's progress during the field experience.

The preceptor needs to be concerned with the schedule of the student. Although some of this responsibility may be delegated to the resident or intern, the preceptor needs to oversee it. The preceptor also needs to ensure that there is physical space for the student and other things which are needed such as identification, a parking permit, and supplies.

Generally, field placements need to contain three elements if they are to be successful. First, the student needs a general orientation to the organization. This may be the same as that given to new employees or it may differ, but it needs to introduce the student to the major physical aspects of the environment as well as to key people and important documents.

Second, the intern or resident needs to spend some time more or less at the elbow of the preceptor, observing the preceptor carry out the hundreds of tasks administrators perform. Major functional areas of planning, organizing, controlling, and evaluating should be represented in the activities which the student observes. This is the time during which a preceptor does the greatest amount of teaching of the student.

Third, the intern or resident needs to have independent work to do, whether projects or some ongoing responsibility. Projects may involve updating the policies and procedures or personnel manuals, development of control systems, or special planning projects. Such independent work is crucial for a number of reasons. It gives the student a chance to work independently, thereby providing an opportunity to try out various administrative functions and roles. It also gives the student something to do when the preceptor is not available and frees the preceptor from the constant need to be thinking about what the student should be doing.

Preceptors should help the students to work out realistic goals for the field experience and should work with the student to develop a schedule for the time the student is in the placement. Over the course of the internship or residency, preceptors should also help students develop short- and long-term career objectives and strategies for obtaining them.

Preceptors need to complete the evaluation documents required and should discuss the evaluation with the student. If, as is recommended, the preceptor is meeting with the student regularly, the evaluation should not be a surprise to the student. Preceptors should also cooperate with faculty supervisors and be available to them.

The Responsibility of the Student in the Field Experience

The role of the intern or resident is a difficult one because it is unfamiliar and singular. The student who becomes an intern or resident has never been one before and has probably had no opportunity to observe anyone else in that role. There are few, if any, similar positions within the organizations where students are placed, so there are no peers to assist in learning the role.

An intern or resident is often in a position within the organization where it is difficult to develop relationships with anyone other than the preceptor. An administrative intern or resident is usually of an age similar to others who are at entry- or middle-level jobs. The intern or resident works at the highest levels of the organization. This disparity between the status due because of age and the status due because of position in the organization may present difficulties to the intern or resident as well as to others in the organization who, being unclear as to how to deal with the student, may choose to ignore him or her.

The separation of an intern from others of a similar age within the organization may leave the student without friends within the organization; this may be particularly difficult for students who are removed physically from their school and need to make friends in a new environment and location. Because of their age, interns and residents may find that some within the organization confide in them — often with things they would rather or should not know. At the same time, the intern or resident may be seen as a spy of top management and shunned by some in the organization.

Interns and residents have an obligation to behave professionally. They need to be responsible and helpful, purposeful and discrete. They need to dress and speak professionally. Students need to be appreciative of the efforts of the preceptor and organization in providing a positive placement experience.

Interns and residents have an obligation to try to obtain maximum benefit from the field experience and to try as hard as possible to make it successful. Students also have an obligation to work with the preceptor to deal with any problem arising in the field and to notify faculty of any problems which remain unresolved.

Students must be responsible about completing assignments for both preceptors and faculty, including reports. They will probably be asked to develop goals and a plan for their time in the field. They will usually be asked to evaluate the placement, and this should be done as objectively as possible.

In some cases students may develop an ongoing close relationship with their preceptor; in others the relationship may be formal and professional. Regardless of the style of the placement, students should express to the preceptor their appreciation for the time and effort expended on them and should remember that no one is obligated to take a student.

Students also have an obligation to leave a placement, even one which they consider has not been a success, in such a manner that the placement can be used again by the program if it seems appropriate.

The student field practicum is often seen as a highlight in the life of a health services administrator. The great majority of them are successful due to the hard work and good will of the student, the educational program and faculty, and the placement preceptor and organization.

REFERENCE

1. Oesterling, *Guidelines for Conducting an Administrator-in-Training Program;* Association of University Programs in Health Administration, *Guidelines for a Clinical/Administrator-in-Training Experience.*

Chapter 6

The Profession

Professionals are defined by six characteristics (1). Measuring Health Services Administration against these criteria is useful for assessing the field and leads to an agenda for the future.

PROFESSIONAL CHARACTERISTICS

Formal Education and Examination

A large percentage of those who are engaged in the administration of health services have not received formal training in the field. This fact, combined with the lack of required examination for any administrators other than those in nursing homes, means that it is very difficult to define who is or is not a health services administrator.

Further complicating the definition is the wide range of organizations in which health services administrators work. These include acute, mental, chronic, and rehabilitation hospitals; long-term care facilities; mental health agencies or clinics; ambulatory care organizations such as community health centers; voluntary associations such as those devoted to birth defects, heart disease, or cancer; hospices; Health Maintenance Organizations (HMOs); and those providing nursing services or health aides in the home.

Although some individual professional societies offer examinations, as noted below, there are no examinations for health services administrators as a group. There may be questions as to whether such an examination would be practicable, but examination, for which the best preparation is education in a carefully designed program, would go far to unify the field and those in it.

A Body of Systematic Scientific Knowledge and Technical Skills

Because of the eclectic nature of Health Services Administration, which integrates knowledge from a number of fields, there has been only partial development of the unique aspects of the field. AUPHA, among others, has given considerable attention to this concern, and its task forces, model curricula, and publications are beginning to demarcate areas of integration. Increasing emphasis on Health Services Research will also encourage definition of the unique knowledge and skills of the field.

The Health Administration Press has an excellent and growing list of book publications which helps to define the field of health administration, and other publishers, such as Aspen, offer publications unique to Health Services Administration.

Health services administrators will have to fend off the efforts of members of other groups to encroach upon the area of Health Services Administration. One such threat comes from physicians who, as the supply of physicians increases to a point of excess in some areas of the country, may find administration attractive. Another source of competition is financial specialists applying their general finance expertise to health care organizations. Of course, there is room for both physicians and financial experts, but not in positions where the integrated knowledge and skills of individuals trained in Health Services Administration would be better.

As financial constraints grow and the demand for efficient and effective delivery of health services also grows, the particular blend of knowledge and skill possessed by the health services administrator may be better appreciated.

Leaders within the field are aware of problems in the area of identification and definition and are working to correct them.

Professional Societies and Associations

Professional societies and associations are the third hallmark of a profession (2). Because of the rapid evolution and development of Health Services Administration, it is particularly important that health services administrators participate in professional groups. Membership and participation improve the practice of the member and thus result in more effective and efficient service delivery. Services offered by these organizations may include workshops, seminars, research sponsorship, and publications.

There are three general types of associations to which health services administrators belong. The first are general interest health organizations. Administrators may be members of the American Public Health Association, which has a Health Administration section, and the affiliated state organizations. Administrators may also belong to organizations which focus on specific aspects of their role such as the American Health Planning Association, or on the population which they serve such as the Gerontology Society. Administrators often belong to local health organizations and to consumer-oriented groups whose primary mission is advocacy for more or better health services.

A second type of association to which administrators belong centers on the organization in which the administrator works. In these, the administrator is not an individual member, but represents his/her facility or agency. Among the best known of these are the American Hospital Association and its state, regional, and district affiliates; the American Association of Homes for the Aging (nonprofit); the American Health Care Association (proprietary nursing homes); and the National Association of Home Care. All of these have state affiliates, and some have regional and district organizations as well.

The third type of association, and perhaps the most important for many administrators, is that associated with the administrator's position. The major groups of this type are described below.

American College of Hospital Administrators, 840 North Lake Shore Drive, Chicago, Illinois 60611.

The primary concerns of the College, founded in 1933, are the development and maintenance of professional standards. Its mission is now defined to include all health administrators rather than just those who work in hospitals.

The College is governed by a Board of Governors. A Council of Regents, elected by membership in the states and in the Canadian provinces, is the legislative arm of the College. There is a committee structure focused on the College's activities in six major areas: Liaison, Membership Services, Education, Project Development and Special Studies, Finance and Operations, and Publications (3).

There are three main types of memberships: nominee for people just beginning careers in Health Administration; membership, for which candidates must take written and oral examinations; and fellowship, which recognizes professional growth and development above and beyond expectations (4). Student associate memberships are also available.

American College of Nursing Home Administrators, P.O. Box 5890, Bethesda, Maryland 20814.

The American College of Nursing Home Administrators, founded in 1962, is pledged to support the development and maintenance of standards and quality among nursing home administrators and the advancement of care for patients, residents, and clients. The major elements in the College's program include publications, *The Long-Term Care Administrator* and *The Journal of Long-Term Care Administration;* a professional referral service; education programs, insurance, and loan programs for members; advocacy for the views of administrators; and a library reference and information service (5).

Anyone "qualified, by training or experience, to engage in the practice of nursing home administration" may become an active member of the College. To become a Fellow, one must have been a member in good standing for at least two years and demonstrated "initiative, leadership, professional growth, and development above and beyond the minimum membership requirements." Members or Fellows can become certified by completing a certification competency assessment workshop and meeting other criteria established by the Professional Certification Committee.

Individuals who are interested in long-term care but are not actively engaged in the administration of a nursing home can become associate members, and there are student and faculty memberships available.

The College is governed by an elected Executive Committee and Board of Governors. The College is divided into twelve regions and forty-seven chapters, corresponding roughly to states or clusters of states. Each member of the College must also belong to a chapter.

Fees are charged for membership applications and for chapter dues. Student memberships are available at a reduced rate.

Healthcare Financial Management Association, 1900 Spring Road, Suite 500, Oak Brook, Illinois 60521 (formerly the Hospital Financial Management Association).

Those engaged in the financial management of health care institutions first organized in 1946. In 1956 this group incorporated as the American Association of Hospital Accountants. In 1968 the name Hospital Financial Management Association was adopted, and in 1982–83 the name was changed to Healthcare Financial Management Association (6).

The Association provides membership services, including training and education; presentations on financial issues in health care to the Health Care Finance Administration, to Congress, and to other associations and the public; and publishes material pertaining to the financial management of health care institutions, including the journal, *Healthcare Financial Management.*

The Association has a matrix organization with councils on Professional Development, Membership and Chapter Services, Professional Excellence, Publications and Communications, and Professional Affairs. Advisory committees deal with Institutions, Corporate Structures, Professional Specialities, Geographic and International, Non-Institutional, and Service Capacity. Overlapping memberships ensure integration among the councils and committees (7).

The Association provides information on and works to improve the financing of health care. Issues with which it has been concerned include uniform billing and Medicare regulations.

Medical Group Management Association, 4101 East Louisiana Avenue, Denver, Colorado 80222.

The Association, founded in 1926, is dedicated to high standards in group practice management. It offers a variety of educational programs for its members, including 200 cassette tapes and independent study courses.

Active membership in the organization is tied to medical group membership. No one can become an active member whose group has not joined. To become a member, an individual's job must involve management responsibility in more than one functional area. Those whose management responsibility is in one functional area may join as associate members provided that their group is a member. Allied membership is open to students, faculty, or those who are managers in groups which do not qualify as members of the Association.

Group dues are based on the number of physicians in the group. There are individual dues and an application fee. Those who are not eligible for membership may join the Correspondent Subscription Service of the Association and receive the journal, monthly newsletter, directory, publication and educational program information, and discounts on some services.

The major publications of the Association are the bimonthly journal, *Medical Group Management*, and *The International Directory*, which is taken from the Association's computerized membership data base. The Association provides an Information Service and conducts a monthly Information Exchange in which members respond to questions on a variety of subjects, thus building a data base. The Association also produces a number of bibliographies and *The Administrator's Bookshelf*, a list of books useful for medical group management.

The Association also provides consulting and placement services for its members and an insurance program. The Association is affiliated with the Center for Research in Ambulatory Health Care Administration, which has received a number of grants for research and demonstration projects.

The Medical Group Management Association participates in the Accreditation Association for Ambulatory Health Care which accredits ambulatory care organizations, including medical group practices.

American Academy of Medical Administrators, Congress Building, 30555 Southfield Road, Suite 525, Southfield, Michigan, 48076.

The American Academy of Medical Administrators (AAMA) was formed in 1957 to meet the need for an organization to serve executive and middle management. Part of the Academy's approach was ". . . based on the theory that the scope of knowledge required to understand an organization and to make it function effectively is based on several fields of knowledge and that approaches to a general theory of medical administration have been slow in emerging. . ." (8). The Academy also works to maximize patient care in a cost-effective manner by supporting management and government working together (9).

Anyone who has been employed in Health Care Administration or Health Care Education for more than two years is eligible to become a nominee. After one year as a nominee, an individual may become a member, and after four years, one becomes eligible to become a Fellow, which also requires the completion of a Project.

The AAMA carries out continuing education activities, publishes "The AAMA Medical Administrative Executive," and annually awards The Charles U. Letourneau Award for the best paper submitted by a graduate student in Health Services Administration. The Academy also awards Honorary Fellowships, a Health Care Executive of the Year Award, and other honors.

Student memberships are available at a nominal fee, and student members receive 75% discounts for conferences and seminars sponsored by the Academy.

Other professional and health-related organizations of interest are listed in Appendix I.

Certification or Licensure

A fourth characteristic of a profession is that certification or licensure is required. This reflects sanction or approval by either the state or a professional body. Certification or licensure may be tied to completion of an approved educational program and/or passage of an examination.

Generally, health services administrators are not required to be licensed or certified. The one exception is that nursing home administrators are required to be licensed. Broad qualifications for administrators, particularly Chief Executive Officers or Executive Directors, may be set by the Joint Commission on Accreditation of Hospitals (JCAH) or by Medicare certification requirements.

Code of Ethics

The best known code of ethics in the health professions is the Hippocratic Oath of physicians. There is no ethical code for health services administrators, although some of the professional societies or associations have one. There is, however, increasing emphasis on ethical concerns in the delivery of health care services, and an increasing number of educational programs offer courses in ethics.

Autonomy and Authority

Because of the special knowledge and skills which a professional is presumed to have, the professionals are given considerable autonomy and authority in their work. Their knowledge and skills are unique to their profession. This means that a professional cannot be judged by someone who is not a peer. A physician, because of the special knowledge and skill she/he has, cannot be judged by a non-physician. The interest of the public and of the patients is protected by the professionals' adherence to the code of ethics, which puts the interest of the patient before that of the doctor. Without the code of ethics, the patient would be at risk. Without the special skill or knowledge, there would be no need for the autonomy, for others could judge or control the work of the professional.

Health services administrators have specialized skill and knowledge. They do not have a code of ethics. Nevertheless, administrators have considerable authority, much of it delegated by the boards of the corporations for which they work. As the boards generally retain the responsibility for the administrator's actions as well as the power to retain or dismiss the administrator, the authority is restricted. Health services administrators are, in fact, constrained as much by law, regulation, and reimbursement requirements as they are by their corporation boards.

In most proprietary situations the administrator stands to profit from his/her actions. There has not been a full discussion of the ethical implications of this within the field, and the importance of clear-cut guidelines for ethical behavior has not been viewed from this perspective. As the for-profit sector of the health care system grows, this deserves additional attention.

THE FUTURE OF HEALTH SERVICES ADMINISTRATION

While it may seem totally obvious to those within the field that trained administrators represent an important element in the delivery of efficient and effective health care services, this does not appear to be universally recognized. The profession faces a number of challenges in the years ahead.

The first challenge is the lack of development and unity in the field. The image of a health services administrator is not clear-cut, and there is no one path to becoming a health services administrator. Some administrators have had no formal educational training at all. Health services administrators are trained in business or management schools, in schools of allied health, schools of medicine, schools of public administration, and schools of public health. The arrangements are usually dependent on variations within individual universities.

Health services administrators, with the exception of nursing home administrators, are not licensed. Licensure, particularly with an examination, might lend unity to a diverse group and prevent those without proper qualifications from entering the field.

It might be argued that accreditation of educational programs would, over time, raise standards and provide sufficient unity within a diverse field. However, many programs cannot meet the accrediting requirements, and the criteria for accreditation may not be relevant to the training of all health services administrators or for all types of positions in all types of organizations.

The fact that both graduate and undergraduate programs are training health services administrators has led to some confusion.

In some parts of the country baccalaureate education in Health Services Administration represents a great leap forward, while in more populous areas, particularly on the east and west coasts, the master's degree is becoming entry-level. While surveys have shown that the great majority of health services administrators have not had formal education in the field, people with newly obtained master's degrees may be unable to find employment. This issue of distribution must be addressed.

Another issue facing the profession is the definition of who is being trained for what. At one time, programs in Hospital Administration aimed to turn out Chief Executive Officers of acute-care hospitals. There is now recognition that fiscal officers, planners, marketers, administrators of nursing, Directors of Materials Management and others need advanced and specialized training. There is also increasing attention given to the need for qualified health services administrators in areas of the health system other than acute care. But leadership within the field is still dominated by the acute-care sector, which also has the bulk of the resources.

Health Services Administration takes knowledge and skills from other disciplines and applies them to the health care system. One result of this is that the field is not evenly developed.

Cost containment pressures have encouraged the development of considerable expertise in the financial management of health care institutions. Through AUPHA and its Task Force on Financial Management Education, this expertise has become widely available.

Health Services Research is in its infancy, although receiving increasing attention. There needs to be increased research in testing the effects of application of knowledge from other fields. There are some examples of areas in which this has been done. The work of Warner and Luce (50) on the applications of cost-benefit and cost-effectiveness analysis to health care is one example. In other areas, for example, employee motivation, little substantive work has been done in applying work from the foundation disciplines to Health Services Administration.

The efficient delivery of effective health services by the organizations and personnel comprising the health system requires coordination and integration, which are the function of administration. To accomplish what is needed, Health Services Administration, as a field, will need to continue to develop and to better define itself to its members and to others inside and outside of the health care system. Students, educators, and practitioners must share so that each may learn from the others, and the theory and practice of Health Services Administration will improve.

REFERENCES

1. Boyles, Morgan, and McCaulley, *The Health Professionals*, p. 32; and Wilson and Neuhauser, *Health Services*, pp. 61-62.

2. Boissoneau, *Continuing Education in the Health Professions*, p. 2.

3. American College of Hospital Administrators, "A Brief Description."

4. Ibid., p. 13.

5. American College of Nursing Home Administrators, "Membership Application," Bethesda, Md.: n.d.

6. Hospital Financial Management Association, "Student Membership Application," Oak Brook, Ill.: n.d.; and *Healthcare Financial Management*, September, 1982, p. 76.

7. Healthcare Financial Management Association, *Annual Report*, in *Healthcare Financial Management*, September, 1982, p. 7.

8. "The AAMA Medical Administrative Executive," Vol. XIX, No. VI, August, 1982, p. 14.

9. American Academy of Medical Administrators, "Do You Qualify? Reach Your Professional Potential."

Chapter 7

Program Model

This chapter provides illustrations of the major elements of a university-based educational program as described in the previous chapters. A complete program is not given here. What is shown here is: program foundations, sample syllabuses, administrative material supporting the field placement or internship and a variety of evaluation instruments.

As with all curriculum and course material, it is continually being revised and updated. The material presented here is from a small undergraduate program. The material required to support a graduate program, or a larger, more complex undergraduate, would be quite different.

Additionally, the program from which this material came, that at the University of Lowell where the authors are faculty members, is unique, as are all programs. Each has environmental and internal conditions and imperatives which make it different from every other program. This program is in a state university which has defined its mission as serving the people of the region, through teaching, research and community service. Programs in universities with a different mission should reflect that difference.

This program is in a College of Health Professions which has a core curriculum for the first two years. This core curriculum includes Anatomy and Physiology, Microbiology, and Physiological Sciences. The value of these courses to students majoring in Health Services Administration, has been discussed. While these courses replace other courses more directly connected to Health Services Administration, many students have used them to good advantage, securing employment or going on to graduate work in a wide range of related areas. The core curriculum does provide students within the College of Health Professions with the opportunity to reassess their choice of major during their freshman and sophomore years, to change from one major to another without losing an academic year and to interrelate with students from other majors.

This chapter has four sections: Program Foundations, Syllabuses, Internship, and Evaluation. At the beginning of each section there is a brief explanation of the material.

PROGRAM FOUNDATIONS

This section includes program philosophy, program objectives and the Program of Studies or curriculum of a typical program. As discussed in Chapter 4, these are sequential with each drawn from the work preceding.

Philosophy

The faculty of the program in Health Services Administration believes that individuals are unique, rational human beings who respond to a changing environment on the basis of essential needs and values. Individuals have an innate right to optimal health. Health Services Administration professionals strive to facilitate the delivery to each individual, in a dignified manner, those health and human services necessary to the attainment of an optimal level of health.

The Health Services Administration program is based on both academic and practical competencies. Health Services Administration develops and refines its specific foundations of knowledge and uses these to continually expand both theory and practice.

As practitioners in a scientific discipline, the health services administrator works with other health professionals to create holistic service modalities, assisting individuals, groups and communities to meet health needs. Health Services Administrators are self-directed decision-making, goal-oriented practitioners and must be able to use knowledge from the fields of management, law, clinical sciences, behavioral sciences, computer sciences, statistics and research methods.

The program in Health Services Administration will prepare competent, entry-level professionals practicing in a variety of settings, who have a foundation for continued personal and professional growth and development.

Objectives

The recipient of the Bachelor of Science in Health Services Administration will:

1. Utilize a broad-based body of knowledge encompassing the biological and social sciences to promote the optimal health of the individual.

2. Identify the major interrelated components, elements, and issues which affect the organization and delivery of contemporary health care services in a changing environment.

3. Describe the relationship of sociocultural, ethical and moral influences on the behavior of health care consumers, professionals, providers and government agencies.

4. Apply knowledge of the legal, fiscal, legislative and environmental factors influencing health care and its delivery.

5. Apply administrative and management principles and techniques as they relate to goal setting, planning, implementation, and evaluation within the organizational structures of health care.

6. Exhibit entry-level skills in administration and management practice including human relations and communication abilities.

7. Recognize the need for continued personal and professional growth.

8. Fulfill the University and departmental criteria for full completion of the academic and clinical program in Health Services Administration.

Course of Study for Health Services Administration

Fall Semester		Spring Semester	
Intro. to Health Prof.	2	Community Health	3
Anatomy & Physiology I.	3	Anatomy & Physiology II	3
Anatomy & Physiology Lab I.	1	Anatomy & Physiology Lab II	1
College Writing	3	College Writing & Lit..	3
Psychology Elective	3	Physical Education	1
Sociology Elective	3	Elective, Area II	3
Physical Education	1	Elective	3
	16		17

Fall Semester		Spring Semester	
Contemp. Health Problems	3	Intro. to Gerontology.	3
Basic Clin. Microbiology & Path.	3	Physiologic Science II.	3
Basic Clin. Microbio. & Path. Lab	1	Physiologic Science Lab II.	1
Physiologic Science I	3	Basic Programming I	3
Physiologic Science Lab I	1	Accounting Principles II	3
Accounting Principles I.	3	Economics II	3
Elective, Area II	3		16
	17		

Fall Semester		Spring Semester	
Long Term Care	3	Dynamics of Interpersonal Rel.	3
Health Care Finance I.	3	Health Care Finance II	3
Sociology of Health	3	Health Planning & Policy	3
Intro. to Statistics	3	Organizational Behavior	3
Computer Elective	3	Elective (Major Area)	3
	15	Elective	3
			18

Fall Semester		Spring Semester	
Health Law & Regulation	3	Program Development, Management & Evaluation	3
Trends in Mental Health	3	Admin. Internship in HSA II	9
Admin. Internship in HSA I.	6	Advanced Seminar in HSA	3
Admin. Seminar in HSA I	3		
	15		15

SYLLABUSES

Four sample syllabuses are shown here for professional courses within the Health Services Administration program. These four illustrate the variety of concerns in curriculum development and revision.

The course in Health Planning and Policy is taught in the second semester of the junior year. Until three years ago it had been taught in the senior year, but faculty felt that it was necessary for students to have this course before beginning their internship, particularly since at least one student usually went to a Health Systems Agency.

This course has been revised repeatedly, partly because of a change in faculty and partly because of the rapid changes taking place in the field. This is perhaps the most overloaded course in the program of studies, and it is clear that the next curriculum revision would have to redistribute some of this material.

In practice, this course is taught by the same faculty member who teaches Health Law and Regulation, and the study of policy in this semester, therefore, feeds well into the study of law and regulation. Students in the course of a year are thus able to see how policy is developed, is converted into law and regulation, and finally into policies and procedures within individual organizations and institutions.

The course in Health Law and Regulation does not attempt to teach case law per se, although the course cases are studied. The aim of the course is to acquaint students with the implications of health law and regulation for them as practicing health services administrators. It therefore stresses how laws and regulations are made, how administrators can keep track of what is happening in the field, and the importance of professional societies and associations in tracking and influencing these developments.

Major areas of health law are dealt with in terms of their effect on administrative practice, but students are cautioned on the changing areas of the law. Because some students have not had Business Law, which can be taken as an elective, some time is spent on contracts. This has been one of the best-liked courses in the curriculum because students feel that the material is relatively discrete and concrete, and because they glimpse the worlds that are being opened to them. The course seems to clarify a great deal that they observe in their internship.

This course is paired with another and is taught six hours a week for one-half semester.

The other two syllabuses are from the year long administrative seminar. Basic work on administrators and administration is included in these courses in lieu of earlier course work defining the field. Personnel administration is covered to some extent. Students have had a course in Organizational Behavior so in the seminar the work is more concrete. It is hoped that the student's knowledge of recruitment, interviewing, job analysis and description, salaries and wages will help them when they are job hunting. This fits well with the emphasis in the seminar on students' planning to meet their personal goals.

The seminars also include a section on the client/patient perspective.

Other material to be covered is less strictly defined. Because the program is small, the faculty usually assesses each class's areas of interest or need and consults with students. Material has varied because of changes in faculty, changes in the program of study, electives taken by the students, and the students' aspirations and interests.

A large portion of the work in the seminars is accomplished through the use of cases. There is an attempt to find or develop cases requiring integration of knowledge and skills from previous courses.

The flexibility which has resulted from the ability of faculty to decide on additional material to be included according to the individual students has worked well and has allowed the program to make maximum use of faculty strengths while providing students with the opportunity to strengthen perceived weaknesses and develop in specific areas of interest.

These four syllabuses illustrate four courses which contribute in a major way to the development of health services administrators. Each year the syllabuses have been revised, and they accurately reflect the strengths and dilemmas faced by a particular program in the areas of curriculum and course design.

Syllabus I

I. Title: 32-411 Health Law and Regulation

II. Course Description:

This course provides the students with a study of the laws and regulations that affect health care and the delivery of health services.

III. Course Objectives:

At the completion of this course the students will be able to:

A. Describe how federal and state laws are made, comparing reality to the idealized process.

B. Explain how regulations are developed and implemented by federal and state governments.

C. Describe the role of local government in protecting the health of the community.

D. Demonstrate the effect of federal and state regulations on the administration of health care organizations.

E. Define and explain legal terms and principles including: contracts, tort law, liability, informed consent, malpractice, and patients' rights.

F. Analyze the ways in which a health services administrator is guided and constrained by legal principles.

G. Design administrative policies and procedures which will prevent lawsuits and minimize risk.

IV. General Information:

A. Time allotment: 3 class hours, 3 credit hours

B. Placement–Course is open to seniors in Health Services Administration and to Health Minors.

C. Attendance. Because of the scheduling of this course, a great deal of material will be covered in each class session. Much of the material discussed in class is not available in the texts. It is, therefore, imperative that students attend each class. For each class missed, students will be given the equivalent of an F for 1% of their total final grade. Students are asked to notify the instructor in advance of class if they are to be absent.

D. Office Hours (Weed 324): Wednesday, 10:00-11:00 and 1:00-2:00; Thursday, 4:00-5:00; Or by appointment.

E. Teaching Methods:
   1. Lectures
   2. Guest speakers
   3. Field trips
   4. Guided library research
   5. Group work
   6. Projects

F. Evaluation Methods

Mid Term.	.20%
First Report	.20%
Second Report . . .	.20%
Final Exam	.40%
	100%

V. Course Requirements:

A. Students are responsible for attending class on a regular basis as described in IV, C.

B. Students are responsible for the readings shown on the course outline attached and any others which may be assigned in class.

C. Mid-Term Examination.

D. First Report. Each student is to take one section of federal or state regulations and describe briefly how they affect some activity which is observed in the student's internship. Students may find it useful to look at established policies and procedures in the relevant area. Please include in the report the relevant section of regulations, giving the citation correctly.

   These reports will be judged on:
   1. Student's choice of topic
   2. Student's ability to show a direct relationship between the regulations and the activity.
   3. The degree to which the form of the report assists the reader in understanding the content.
   4. Overall presentation.

E. Second Report. Students are to write or revise a set of policies and if appropriate the procedures to implement them. Students may do this report in partnership with one other student.

   Students should use as the basis for the policies, one of the following:
   1. Federal or state regulations. Use one section only.
   2. JCAH, Medicare, or state criteria

   Students may write policies for a specific organization, for example the one in which their internship is being done, or for a hypothetical organization which they define.

   If regulations are used, relevant section of the regulations should be included and a correct citation given. If other standards are used as the basis for the policies, the standards should be given.

These reports will be judged on:
1. Choice of topic
2. Student's ability to interpret the regulation or criteria
3. Clarity and lack of ambiguity of policies and procedures
4. Overall presentation

F. Final Examination

VI. Required Texts:
1. Pozgar, George D.: *Legal Aspects of Health Care Administration*, 2nd Edition, Rockville, MD: Aspen, 1983.
2. Annas, George J.: *The Rights of Hospital Patients* (An American Civil Liberties Union Handbook), New York: Avon Books, 1975.
3. Conservation Law Foundation of New England, Inc.: *Legal Handbook for Boards of Health.* Boston, MA, 1982.

VII. Other:

A. Policy on Make-Up Examinations. Under normal circumstances, make-up examinations will not be given. Under no circumstances will a make-up examination be provided for any student who does not notify the instructor before the examination of his or her inability to take it. The judgment of whether or not a make-up examination will be given is solely that of the instructor. Any make-up examination provided will be considerably more difficult than that given at the scheculed time.

B. Penalties for Late Reports. Reports which are submitted after the dates indicated will be penalized ½ of a full grade for each class day the report is late.

C. Confidentiality. It is possible that during the course, the instructor, guest speakers, or students in the class will wish to share information having to do with specific organizations or individuals. Such information should be treated as confidential and not discussed outside of the classroom. Students in their internships will be bound by the same laws of privacy and confidentiality as other health professionals. If students are in doubt as to whether or not they may share something in the class, or take from the class specific information, they should consult the instructor.

NOTE: "All students are advised that there is a University policy regarding dishonesty and cheating. It is the students' responsibility to familiarize themselves with the policies." If necessary, contact your advisors or instructors for clarification of these policies.

7/8/83

Course Outline

32-411 Health Law and Regulations

Oct. 26 Introduction to Course and Introduction to Law
Pozgar: Chapter
Annas: Appendix C

Oct. 28 Federal Government

Oct. 31	Field Trip to Government Documents
Nov. 2 &	State Government
Nov. 4	Legal Handbook: pp. 1–10 (through Part A)
	Pozgar: Chapter 8
Nov. 7	Field Trip to State House
Nov. 9	Local Government: Guest Speaker
	Legal Handbook: pp. 10–24
Nov. 14 &	Torts and Contracts
Nov. 16	Pozgar: Chapters 1, 2, 15
Nov. 18	MID-TERM
Nov. 21	Liability (and Malpractice)
	Pozgar: Chapters 3, 4, 5, 14
Nov. 23	Organizational Governance
	Annas: Chapter 11
	Pozgar: Chapter 3
Nov. 28	FIRST REPORT DUE
	Physician-Patient Relationships
	Pozgar: Chapters 4 (Review), 6, 12
	Annas: Chapters VI, VII, VIII, XVII, XVIII
Nov. 30	Hospital-Patient Relationships
	Annas: Chapters III, IV, V, X, Appendix D
Dec. 2	Hospital Records and Privacy
	Pozgar: Chapter 7
	Annas: Chapters X, XI
Dec. 5	Informed Consent
	Pozgar: Chapters 6, 10
	Annas: Chapters VI, IX
Dec. 7	Labor Law
	Pozgar: Chapter 13
Dec. 9	Reproductive Issues: Abortion, Sterilization, Artificial Insemination, Genetic Screening, RDNA
	Pozgar: Chapters 9, 11
	Annas: Chapter XIII
Dec. 12	SECOND PROJECT DUE
	Issues of Death, Dying, and Treating the Terminally Ill Patient
	Pozgar: Chapter 10, Appendix A
	Annas: Chapter XIV
Dec. 14	Review and Evaluation

Syllabus II

I. Title: 32-422 Health Planning and Policy

II. Course Description:

Traces the historical development of major national and state health policies and provides practice in applying a framework for policy analysis. Examines the history of population-based health planning and the current status of Health Systems Agencies. Emphasizes strategic planning in health care organizations and provides practice in elements of the planning process. Includes a survey of major marketing principles and their application to health care organizations.

III. Course Objectives:

At the completion of this course, the student will be able to:

A. Describe major federal and state health policy issues and the philosophical bases of prescribed solutions.
B. Compare the effectiveness of health policy efforts, identifying factors contributing to or preventing successful implementation.
C. Analyze a specific federal or state policy, using or adapting a prescribed methodology.
D. Trace the development of population-based and strategic planning.
E. Compare population-based and strategic planning.
F. Identify and describe data available to the community or institutional planner.
G. Identify information sources available to the health planner.
H. Use quantitative techniques appropriate to the planning process.
I. Identify the major principles of marketing health services.
J. Communicate more effectively and present material in non-verbal ways.
K. Describe the role of the health services administrator in planning and marketing.

IV. General Information:

A. Time allotment: 3 class hours, 3 credit hours
B. Placement: HSA junior only
C. Attendance. Regular attendance is required. More than three absences will be considered excessive.
D. Office Hours (Weed Hall, Room 324): Monday, 10:00-11:00; Friday, 9:00-10:00 and 12:00-1:00
E. Teaching methods:
   1. Lectures
   2. Guest speakers
   3. Group work
   4. Class Discussion
   5. Assigned problems
   6. Paper
   7. Readings
   8. Field trip
F. Evaluation methods:

Participation	10%
Problems 3 (15% each)	45%
Paper (Oral 10%, Written 10%)	20%
Final Exam	25%
	100%

V. Course Requirements:

A. Attendance. Regular attendance is required as discussed in Section IV, C.

B. Problems. 3 problems will be assigned. They are due on February 22, March 14, and April 18.

C. Paper.

1. Students will prepare a paper on a major state or national health policy. Analysis will be done using the framework distributed and discussed in class. The topic must be approved by the instructor.
2. This paper is due on April 30, and must be in approved form. Late papers will be penalized heavily.
3. Students will also do an oral presentation of this paper. The presentation is limited to 15 milutes.

D. Final Examination. The final examination will be given at the time assigned by the Registrar.

VI. Required Texts:

A. Thompson, Frank J.: *Health Policy and the Bureaucracy: Politics and Implementation.*

B. Altman, Drew; Green, Richard; and Sapolsky, Harvey: *Health Planning and Regulation: The Decision-Making Process.*

C. American Hospital Association. *Strategic Thinking.*

VII. Other:

Make-up Examination. A make-up examination will be given only if there is good cause and the student notifies the instructor before the start of the examination. The decision as to whether a make-up examination will be given is solely the instructor's.

NOTE: "All students are advised that there is a university policy regarding dishonesty and cheating. It is the student's responsibility to familiarize themselves with these policies. If necessary, contact your advisors or instructors for clarification of these policies."

Course Outline

Jan. 23	Introduction to Course
Jan. 25	Health Policy — An Overview Thompson: Chapters 1, 8
Jan. 27	Defining Death President's Commission for the Study of Ethical Problems in Medicine and Biomedical and Behavioral Research, *Deciding to Forego Life-Sustaining Treatment* Chapter 1, pp. 15-41 (on reserve)
Jan. 30 & Feb. 1	Cost containment, quality and access Altman: Chapter 1 Thompson: Chapter 3
Feb. 3 & Feb. 6	Medicare and Medicaid as Public Policy Thompson: Chapters 3, 4

Feb. 8	Community Health Centers
	Thompson: Chapter 3
Feb. 10 &	Citizen Participation
Feb. 13	Altman: Chapters 4 and 3, Cases 6, 7
	Ellenburg: "Special Interests vs. Citizen Control" (on reserve)
Feb. 15	Community Mental Health
Feb. 17 &	Technology Assessment and Ethical Choices
Feb. 21	Altman: Chapter 7, Case 8 Force
	Final Report of the Task on Liver Transplantation in Massachusetts (on reserve)
Feb. 22	*Comprehensive Health Planning*, PROBLEM No. 1 DUE
Feb. 24 &	P.L. 93-641, and Health Systems Agencies
Feb. 27	Thompson: Chapter 2
	HSA IV, Application for Renewal of Designation as Health Systems Agency (on reserve)
Feb. 29	Sources of Data
	Reading on reserve in Library
Mar. 2	Guidelines and Standards
	Altman: Case 2, Chapter 6
Mar. 5	Analytical techniques: Bed Need Methodology
Mar. 7	Small Area Analysis
Mar. 9 &	Determination of Need
Mar. 12	DON Applications on reserve in Library
Mar. 14 &	PROBLEM No. 2 DUE
Mar. 16	Development and Implementation of Plans and Projects
	Altman: Chapter 5, Case 3
	HPCGB, Health Systems Plan, IV (on reserve, browse through it)
	Report of the Community Hospital Planning Committee (on reserve)
SPRING VACATION	
Mar. 16	Institutional Planning
	Strategic Thinking: pp. 95-96
Mar. 28 &	Strategic Planning
Mar. 30	*Strategic Thinking:* Chapters 1-6
Apr. 2	Developing a Strategic Plan
	Strategic Thinking: Chapters 7, 8, 10
Arp. 4	Market Drives vs. Service Driven Planning
Apr. 6	Medical Staff and Physician Issues
Apr. 9	Strategic Planning for Non-Acute Health Care Organizations
Apr. 11	Role of the Community
Apr. 13	Catch-Up Day
Apr. 18 &	PROBLEM No. 3 DUE
Apr. 20	Principles of Marketing
Apr. 23 &	Marketing Capacity
Apr. 25	

Apr. 30 POLICY ANALYSIS PAPERS DUE
Student Reports on Policy Analysis
May 2
May 4
May 7
May 9 Evaluation and Review
Other Readings may be assigned as necessary

Syllabus III

Fall Semester

I. Title: 32-415 Seminar in Health Services Administration I

II. Course Description:
This seminar will provide students with an understanding of the theory and practice of health services administration and an opportunity to explore the component processes of the management of health services. Students will be required to apply the experiences of their internships and the literature of health services administration to seminar discussion and to problems and case studies emphasizing analytical, evaluative and decision-making skills.

III. Course Objectives:
By the end of this seminar, students will have:
A. Defined health services administration as a profession.
B. Demonstrated knowledge of current theory and practice in health services administration.
C. Identified the responsibilities of the health services administrator.
D. Classified types of administrators and explained the strengths and weaknesses of each type.
E. Identified the components of the administrative role and their application within the internship setting.
G. Developed goals, objectives, strategies, policies and procedures.
H. Proposed and defended solutions to simple administrative problems and cases.
I. Worked effectively in groups assigned specific tasks.
J. Improved their written and oral communication skills.

IV. Course Requirements:
A. Attendance and Participation. The responsibility for the success of the seminar is shared by the instructor and students. Much of the material for this seminar will be drawn from students' observations and activities in their internships. Because each student has a different experience in the internship, each has a responsibility to attend the seminar and participate as appropriate. Students will be expected to improve their ability to communicate orally.
B. Problems. Two brief problems will be assigned. Students will be asked to apply the concepts discussed in the text and in seminar to the internship experience.

C. Case. One case will be assigned. This will be done in groups. The cases require students to analyze the situation presented, suggest alternative solutions, recommend one solution and support that choice.

D. Mid-term. There will be a mid-term which will cover the material on Health Services Administration as a profession, the health care system, and health care organizations. There will be no final exam.

E. Paper.

1. Each student, individually or in groups of up to four, is to write a major paper. While the subject should be related to the internship, the data for this paper should come mainly from the literature, including government documents.
2. Each student or group is to choose a topic which represents an area of activity under the supervision of a health services administrator. The paper should include:
   a. The usual way in which this activity is carried out and supervised.
   b. The relation of the activity to the administrator of the facility or agency.
   c. The changes which are taking place in the way this activity is carried out.
   d. The issues related to this activity which are currently under discussion.
3. The activity which is to be the subject of the paper should be an activity which goes on in some health facilities or organizations. It may be broad or narrow, mundane or more philosophical. Possible topics include: management information systems, laundry, food preparation, fund raising, union negotiations, benefits, bill collection, purchasing or materials management, personnel recruitment, marketing, or a vast array of others.

F. Oral Presentation.

1. The student or group doing each paper will have ten minutes to present their paper. Students will be heavily penalized for exceeding the time limit and are urged to practice before the presentation to be sure that they stay within the limit.
2. If the paper is done by a group, the group may divide up the oral presentation or choose one or more of the members to do the presentation. However, all members of the group will be held responsible for the presentation and all will receive the same grade — whether or not the individual student has done the presentation.
3. The criteria on which the presentation will be graded will be distributed and discussed during class.

V. Requires Readings:

A. The basic text for this course is *Management of Health Services*, by Arnold Kaluzny, D. Michael Warner, David Warren and William

Zelman, Prentice Hall, 1982. We will also be using *The Human Side of Health Administration* by Robert Veninga, Prentice Hall, 1982. This is a paperback, but some of you might wish to share it.

B. You will also be required to read three simple chapters in *The Challenge of Administering Health Services: Career Pathways*, edited by Lowell Bellin and Lewis Weeks, AUPHA Press, 1982. Copies of this are on reserve.

C. Other texts are available in the library.

D. Suggested Readings (reserved in library)

1. Students are expected to use the literature for the problems, paper and case as appropriate. The library has an excellent selection of journals in the field including:
   a. *Health Care Management Review*
   b. *Health Services Manager*
   c. *Health Services Research*
   d. *Hospitals*
2. Students are encouraged to make use of other journals on administration and on health.
3. If a topic is of current interest, preceptors or the agency or facility in which an internship is being done, may have additional, useful material.
4. If students are unable to find enough information, I will be glad to help.

VI. Confidentiality:

Students, faculty and guest speakers will be sharing information and views within the seminar. All such material should be considered confidential and not discussed outside of the seminar. If students have any doubt as to what should be discussed in the seminar, they should seek advice from their internship preceptor, the faculty member supervising their internship or the instructor.

VII. Course Outline

Sept. 8	Organization of course and internship
Sept. 13 &	Health Services Administration
Sept. 15	Kaluzny: Chapters 1, 14
	Veninga: Chapter 1
	Bellin and Weeks: Chapter 1
Sept. 20	Guest Speaker
Sept. 22	The Health Services System
	Kaluzny: Chapter 13
	Bellin and Weeks (on reserve), read 2 chapters from among chapters 2 through 11
Spet. 27	Discussion of internships
Sept. 29 &	Health Services Organizations
Oct. 4	Kaluzny: Chapters 2, 3
	Veninga: Chapter 2
Oct. 6	PROBLEM NO. 1 DUE

	Research Librarian, South Campus
Oct. 13	Administrative Competence
	Veninga: Chapters 3, 4, 6
Oct. 18	Catch-up
Oct. 20	Mid-Term
Oct. 25	Administrative Competence (continued)
Oct. 27	Guest Speaker
Nov. 1	Planning and Budgeting (Introduction)
	Kaluzny: Chapters 4, 5
Nov. 3	Field trip
Nov. 8	PROBLEM NO. 2 DUE
	Planning and Budgeting (continued)
Nov. 10	Governemnt Documents — North Campus
Nov. 15	Planning and Budgeting (continued)
Nov. 17	Field trip
Nov. 22, &	Implementation
Nov. 24 &	Kaluzny: Chapter 6
Nov. 29	
Dec, 1, 6,	Student Presentations
8 & 13	
Dec. 15	Course Evaluation

VIII. Evaluation:

Attendance and Participation. 10%
Mid-Term 20%
Problems (10% each) 20%
Case 15%
Paper — Written Presentation. 25%
Oral Presentation 10%
100%

Syllabus IV

I. Title: Seminar in Health Services Administration II, 32-418

II. Course Description:

Case studies will be used to give students practice in decision-making. There will be considerable emphasis on the administrator's relationship with others in the health care system and with those outside the health care system whose activities impinge upon the administrator. Students will be expected to use their internship experience in the seminar. This seminar taken with Administrative Internship II.

III. Course Objectives:

At the completion of this course, students will have:

A. Analyzed a number of administrative cases and presented alternative solutions in a concise, well-organized form.

B. Practiced interpreting data presented in a variety of ways and acquired basic concepts and skills in the presentation of data.

C. Demonstrated knowledge of major tasks and functions in personnel management in health care organizations.
D. Exhibited an understanding of the patient/client role.
E. Demonstrated improved written and oral communication skills.
F. Developed strategies for reaching personal goals.

IV. General Information:

A. Time allotment: 3 class hours, 3 credit hours
B. Placement. Course is open to seniors in Health Services Administration who are concurrently taking Administrative Internships II.
C. Attendance. The responsibility for the success of the seminar is shared by the instructor and students. Much of the material for the seminar will be drawn from students' observations and activities in their internships and personal skills and knowledge. Because each student brings different experiences to the seminar, particularly from the internship, each student has a responsibility to attend the seminar and participate as appropriate. A student who is not at the seminar obviously cannot participate, and absence will affect the student's final grade.
D. Office Hours: Monday, 10:00-11:00; Friday 9:00-10:00, 12:00-1:00; or by appointment (ext. 2830).
E. Teaching Methods:
   1. Lecture
   2. Guest speakers
   3. Cases
   4. Group work
   5. Discussion
F. Evaluation Methods

Mid-Term	20%
Participation	10%
Data Assignments	25%
Case Assignments (15% each)	45%
	100%

V. Course Requirements:

A. Students are responsible for attending class on a regular bases as described in Section IV, C.
B. Students are responsible for contributing to the seminar, by participating in class discussion, being prepared to discuss the assigned cases, and as requested by the instructor.
C. Students are responsible for the readings shown on the attached course outline and others which may be assigned in class.
D. Mid-Term Examination: March 14.
E. Data Assignment. Students will be asked to present data generated from a data set on the computer. Details of this assignment will be presented in class. Due April 11.
F. Cases. Students will be responsible for 3 case analyses, which are to be done following the method discussed in class. One will be done in

a group, one with a partner, and one individually. The individual case will be presented orally, the others will be written. These cases are due Febryary 8, March 7, and April 18.

VI. Required Texts:

A. Norman Metzger, *Personnel Administration in the Health Services Industry*, 2nd Edition.

B. Jonathan S. Rakich, Beaufort B. Longest, Jr., and Kurt Darr, *Cases in Health Services Management.*

C. Erving Goffman, *Asylums* OR Martha Weinman Lear, *Heartsounds.*

VII. Other:

A. Policy and Make-Up Examinations. Under normal circumstances, make-up examinations will not be given. Under *no* circumstances will a make-up examination be provided for any student who does not notify the instructor before the examination of his or her inability to take it. The judgment of whether or not a make-up examination will be given is solely that of the instructor.

B. Penalties for Late Reports. Reports which are submitted after the dates indicated will be penalized one full grade for each class day they are late.

C. Confidentiality. During the course the instructor, guest speakers or students may wish to share information having to do with specific organizations or individuals. Such information should be treated as confidential and not discussed outside of the classroom. Students in their internships will be bound by the same laws of privacy and confidentiality as other health professionals. If students are in doubt as to whether or not they may share something in the class, or take from the class specific information, they should consult the instructor.

D. Cheating. "All students are advised that there is a University policy regarding dishonesty and cheating. It is the students' responsibility to familiarize themselves with these policies." If necessary contact your advisor or instructor for clarification of these policies.

Course Outline

Jan. 25 Resumes
The Effective Administrator
Rakich: Cases 1, 4, 5, 6, 9

Feb. 1 Guest Speaker: Resumes
Interviewing and Networking
The Effective Administrator (II)

Feb. 8 CASE NO. 1 DUE (use 1, 4, 5, and 6, or 9)
Job Analysis and Description; Recruitment, Screening, and Selection
Metzger: Chapters 1, 2, 4

Feb. 15	Job Evaluation and Wage and Salaries Administration, Contract Administration Metzger: Chapters 3, 8 Rakich: Case 30
Feb. 22	Graduates of the Program Rakich: Cases 23, 24, 26, 28
Mar. 7	CASE NO. 2 DUE (Choose from 3, 8, 23, 24, 26, 28) Guest Speaker: Dealing with the Bureaucracy Organizational Governance Rakich: Case, 11, 12, 13, 18, 27
Mar. 14	MID-TERM Job-Hunting Strategies
Mar. 28	Methods of Data Presentation
Apr. 4	Methods of Data Presentation II
Apr. 11	DATA PRESENTATION ASSIGNMENT DUE The Patient/Client Perspective All of Heartsounds or pp. 1-124 of Goffman
Apr. 18	Oral Case Presentations
Apr. 25	Oral Case Presentations
May 2	The Effective Administrator Revisited
May 9	Evaluation and Assessment — Course and Program

Additional readings may be assigned in class.

INTERNSHIP

As discussed in Chapter 5, the internship or residency is a very important part of the professional education of a health service administrator.

Because the university interacts with health care organizations in regard to the field placement, there is considerably more administrative work than with other courses. This is particularly true for undergraduate programs with internships which tend to use active faculty involvement to more carefully monitor students in the field placement.

This section includes the documents and forms which have been found to help the administration of the internship.

The "Guide to the Administrative Internship" lays out the responsibilities of those involved in the internship experience as well as the objectives. This guide is distributed to students and preceptors, and is given to prospective preceptors when they are considering whether or not they wish to be involved with the program.

The next two forms, Information Sheet for Internship Placement and Preference Sheet for HSA Internship Placement are used to gather information about the student and his/her preferences about internship. There is considerable discussion with students before the forms are filled out so that students have realistic expectations and information on which to base their choices.

The syllabuses are intended to complement the guide and to make clear the intern's responsibilities to the university and to the faculty member supervising the internship. Again, there have been changes over the years in these requirements. Generally, students are required to keep a journal during both semesters with entries each day they are at internship during the first semester. This permits faculty to do considerable work with students on writing and to interact more continuously with students, staying in closer touch with what is going on. As the program has matured, it has been found that this intensive writing practice is not necessary in the second semester and students are required to write more thoughtful and analytical entries once a week.

Similarly, it has been found that assignments more closely tied to the internship work better and these assignments, requiring in some cases rather active participation by the preceptor, have met with considerable approval in preceptor evaluations.

To facilitate the internship and to make sure that there is a direction and purpose to the internship, students are required to develop goals and a plan for the internship. A form is provided for the goals; not having a form for the plan allows preceptors and faculty to work with students on the development of a format for the plan.

The Field Visit Form provides a convenient way for having those concerned acknowledge the visit of the faculty supervisor to the placement site. The form enables the faculty member responsible for coordinating the internship to conveniently monitor the field visits.

Three forms are used to evaluate the internship experience at its conclusion. The first is the evaluation of the student done by the preceptors. An attempt is made to ensure that preceptors and interns discuss this evaluation on an ongoing basis, but faculty is not always successful in promoting this.

There is also a form on which preceptors are asked to evaluate their experience with the internship and their dealings with the university. Students are similarly asked to anonymously evaluate their internship experiences.

Guide to the Administrative Internship In Health Services Administration

Introduction

The College of Health Professions offers a major in Health Services Administration in cooperation with the College of Management Science. This program prepares graduates for entry-level positions in hospitals, nursing homes, planning agencies, boards of health, ambulatory care organizations, and other health services providers. The Health Services Administration program has been approved by the Association of University Programs in Health Administration (AUPHA).

An important component of the major in Health Services Administration is the administrative internship in the senior year. Students spend two days a week in their internship fall semester and are in the field two to four days a week during spring semester. A qualified administrator acts as preceptor and provides guidance as the student practices the skills and knowledge acquired in the academic program. A faculty supervisor from the College of Health Professions carries the responsibility for the suitability of placements, supervises the internship and provides assistance to students and preceptors.

Student internships will usually entail rotation through the departments of a health services facility or agency or the assignment of responsibility for a specific project. The exact mix of activity will vary according to the needs of the facility or agency and the ability of a student.

Responsibilities of the Agency or Facility

The agency or facility where the administrative intern is placed shall:

1. Ensure that the preceptor is qualified and is able to aid in the professional development of the student.
2. Provide the student with sufficient orientation and introduction to the organization's staff, rules, regulations, and policies.
3. Provide the necessary physical facilities and equipment for the student intern.
4. Encourage students to meet a wide range of staff within the facility or agency including administrators of major departments and boards of directors.
5. Provide the intern with the documents and records per-

taining to the facility or agency which the intern needs to complete the learning required during the internship experience.

Responsibilities of the Administrative Intern

The administrative intern shall:

1. Exhibit appropriate conduct with regard to attendance, promptness, neatness, preparedness, purposefulness, and discretion.
2. Spend a minimum of sixteen hours a week in the internship (excluding university vacation periods) at times agreed upon with the preceptor.
3. Prepare a set of personal goals in consultation with the preceptor and university faculty supervisor.
4. Develop a plan for the internship in consultation with the preceptor.
5. Carry out the assignments made by the preceptor to the best of his or her ability.
6. Prepare reports for the preceptor and faculty supervisor as required by each.
7. Prepare a paper or other assignment as required by the university supervisor.
8. Participate in periodic conferences with the preceptor and with the university supervisor.
9. Participate in the final evaluation of the internship with both the preceptor and faculty supervisor.
10. Respect the confidential nature of all agency activities. No discussion of agency, facility, client or patient concerns will take place outside this umbrella of confidentiality.

Responsibilities of the Preceptor

The preceptor shall:

1. Help the intern to develop a plan and realistic goals for the administrative internship.
2. Provide opportunities for the student to assume responsibility commensurate with his or her abilities and which will allow for the exercise of a broad range of administrative skills. The faculty supervisor is able to provide suggestions for such activities.
3. Assign the student to activities which will be of some benefit to the facility or agency as well as to the student.
4. Plan regular meetings with the intern which will allow for assessment of past performance and planning for the future.
5. Provide the intern with the opportunity to meet administrators of similar facilities or agencies; key community, govern-

ment, reimbursement, planning, and regulatory officials; and other health professionals.

6. Provide the student with guidance in making realistic career choices and assist the student in meeting those people who may be of help in locating future employment opportunities.

7. Be available for periodic meetings with the faculty supervisor from the university.

8. Evaluate the student on the form provided by the university by the deadline set by the college.

9. Present evidence of registration as a preceptor with the Massachusetts Board of Registration if a nursing home administrator.

10. Supply the university with a current curriculum vita.

Responsibilities of the Faculty of the Department of Health, College of Health Professions

The faculty of the Department of Health, College of Health Professions shall:

1. Provide each student who has satisfactorily completed the required Health Services Administration courses with a placement, or assist those students who wish to find their own placement.

2. Provide a Memorandum of Agreement between the facility or agency where an internship is to be done and the university and to ensure that this memorandum is signed by both parties.

3. Take responsibility for the content of the internship experience as required by university rules and regulations.

4. Ensure that students are adequately prepared to assume the responsibilities of an administrative internship.

5. Provide the students with adequate information about the internship placement and provide the preceptor and agency or facility with information about the student.

6. Help students to work out individual goals and a plan for the internship.

7. Be available and helpful to students and preceptors.

8. Meet with both the preceptor and student regularly and discuss the progress of the internship with them.

9. Provide each preceptor and student with a form to be used in evaluating the student.

10. Evaluate the student giving due weight to the evaluation of the preceptor.

11. Provide one course voucher to each facility or agency which has an administrative intern.

Objectives of the Internship Program

In the course of the administrative internship, the student will, to the extent possible:

1. Complete an experience in a nursing home, hospital or community health agency which is appropriate to the student's career objectives.
2. Learn the requirements and responsibilities of the profession.
3. Make a positive contribution to the facility or agency in which the internship is done.
4. Acquire responsibility commensurate with the student's ability. In the second semester this will usually involve a project or assignment which can be carried out solely by the intern and which requires the use of a variety of administrative skills.
5. Experience a variety of administrative tasks, including but not limited to fiscal management, employee relations, and quality assurance.
6. Learn to work with and write policies and procedures and develop goals and objectives.
7. Attend professional conferences, seminars and meetings of various types to meet those in government, the community and in other agencies and organizations that provide, regulate, plan or pay for health services.
8. Make realistic career choices and have the opportunity to meet or work with people who may be able to help the student locate employment opportunities.
9. Identify sources of information on changes taking place in the need for health services and in their supply and financing.

In addition to these objectives, each student will, in consultation with his or her preceptor and faculty advisor, develop a set of personal goals appropriate to the placement situation and the strengths and weaknesses of the student.

Information Sheet for Internship Placement

Name ______________________________

School address ______________________________

Telephone number at school ______________________

Home address ______________________

Home telephone ______________________

Education:

Work experience:

Relevant volunteer experience:

Hobbies or other interests:

Other responsibilities (e.g., job, family):

Preference Sheet for HSA Internship Program

For University Use Only

Name ______________________

In what type of agency or facility would you like to be placed? Why?

What would be your second choice?

Do you intend to take the nursing home licensure exam?

Do you wish to be placed in the same internship for both semesters or would you like to be placed in two different internships?

What is your hometowm?

Do you have the use of a car to get to your internship?

In what geographical area would you like to be placed?

Is there a particular agency or facility in which you wish to be placed?

What is your approximate grade point average?

How many credits do you expect to take fall semester?

How many credits do you expect to take spring semester?

Is there anything else you would like us to know about you before you are placed?

What do you expect to do after you graduate?

Syllabus I

I. Title: 32–409 Administrative Internship I

II. Course Description:

The description, objectives, requirements and responsibilities of those involved in the internship are described in the "Guide to the Administrative Internship." Each student should have a copy.

III. General Information:

A. Time allotment: 18 class hours, 6 credit hours.

B. Placement. Course is open only to Seniors in Health Services Administration who are concurrently taking 32–415. Fall Semester — Senior Year.

C. Attendance. Students are expected to be in their field placements as scheduled. Preceptors should be notified immediately of any necessary absence and the faculty supervisor should be consulted about any absence of more than one day. Students may be required to make up missed days.

D. Office hours. Office hours for faculty supervising field internships are posted outside Room 324.

E. Teaching Methods:

1. Field work
2. Journals
3. Paper
4. Group discussion

F. Evaluation Methods:

Preceptor's evaluation . . .60%
Paper 20%
Journals. 20%
100%

IV. Course Requirements:

A. Attendance at internship and performance of assigned duties and tasks.

B. Journals. Each student will keep a detailed journal and make an entry for each day of the internship. In this journal, students will record:

1. What he or she has done in the internship.
2. What is happening at the agency or facility.
3. Comments on the administrative style and functioning of the preceptor and other administrators with whom the student interacts.
4. The student's reaction to the above.
5. Suggestions or comments centering on alternative courses of action which might have been more or less effective.

The emphasis in the journals should be on understanding the dynamics of effective administration, describing the way in which the organization works, and examining the relationship of the agency or facility to the external environment and the health care system at large. Questions — many of which have no answers or for which answers will only become apparent later — should be a major part of the journal. To the extent that personal matters (illness, family problems, car trouble) affect the internship, they should be reported.

The journals are a very important part of the internship and contribute to it in the following ways:

1. Force students to examine their own knowledge, behavior, attitudes and emotions in relation to administrative tasks.
2. Encourage students to view their internships objectively.
3. Accustom students to carrying on continual, if unstructured, evaluation of their own work and that of others.
4. Allow the faculty supervisor to be continually informed about the internship, to identify positive and negative aspects of the experience and work to reinforce the positive and change the negative parts of the experience.
5. Facilitate a continuing dialogue between the student and the faculty supervisor which encourages and aids learning.
6. Contributes to the improvement of writing skills.

Journals should be submitted every other week on:

1. September 19
2. October 3
3. October 17
4. October 31
5. November 14
6. November 28
7. December 14

Students should write the journal on loose sheets of paper kept in a lightweight folder. Students can then continue to make entries while the journals are being read by the faculty advisor.

Journals will be graded for promptness, honesty, openness and the student's willingness to identify and examine the difficult issues presented by their internships. Students will be expected to show improvement in their journal entries.

Confidentiality. The journals are confidential between the student and the faculty supervisor. If several students have presented the same problem, it may be discussed in seminar in general terms. If it is judged necessary to discuss with the internship preceptor a problem presented in the journal, the student will be consulted for approval before this is done.

C. Paper. Each student is to analyze a series of meetings which have been attended as part of the internship. Each student is to briefly describe the meetings: the settings, participants and agenda. Include in your analysis at least the following factors:

1. The stated and unstated purposes of the meetings.

2. The leadership style of the person running the meetings.
3. The degree of participation by others at the meetings.
4. The distribution of men and women at the meetings. What conclusions do you draw from this distribution?
5. The rules which governed the meetings. Were they understood by the participants? Were they written or unwritten? How were they conveyed to the participants?
6. Indications that any of the participants had made preparations for the meetings. What were the consequences of the preparations?
7. The satisfaction which participants received from the meetings.
8. The extent to which the purposes were achieved.
9. Suggestions for accomplishing the purposes in a different way.
10. Anything that was interesting or unusual about these meetings.

D. Internship Goals. Each student is expected to develop a set of individual goals for the internship. Students are to discuss their goals with the preceptor and faculty advisor. A form is provided for the goals with space for the preceptor and faculty member to sign. Goals should be submitted by October 13.

E. Plans for Internship. Each student is to develop, in consultation with his or her preceptor, a flexible plan for the internship. A copy of this plan should be submitted to the faculty supervisor by October 13.

V. Required Text:

There are no required texts. Students may be assigned specific, individual readings by preceptors and/or faculty supervisors.

VI. Additional Information:

A. Students in their internships will be bound by the same laws of privacy and confidentiality as other health professionals. If students are in doubt as to whether or not they may discuss something with those outside the placement agency they should consult their preceptor or faculty supervisor.

B. All students are advised that there is a University policy regarding dishonesty and cheating. It is the students' responsibility to familiarize themselves with these policies. If necessary, contact your advisors or instructors for clarification of these policies.

Syllabus II

I. Title: 32-401 Administrative Internship II

II. Course Description:

The description, objectives, requirements and responsibilities of those involved in the administrative internship are described in the "Guide to the Administrative Internship." Each student should have a copy.

III. Course Requirements:

A. Weekly Report Forms. Each student should complete a Weekly Report Form for each week of the internship. It should be placed in the mailbox of the faculty supervisor on Monday of each week (Room 222).

B. Journals

1. The journals should contain the student's questions, comments and musings on the administrative internship. It should generally be written once a week, although additional entries may be warranted under certain circumstances. Students should not attempt to summarize their activities as that will be done on the weekly report form. Rather, students should be offering reactions, interpretations, analysis and questions on what they are observing and thinking.
2. It is not necessary to cover a great number of topics in each journal entry. One topic, discussed in depth, may be sufficient.
3. The following topics are suggested as appropriate for consideration; students are encouraged to consider what is important in relation to the organization in which they have been placed.
   a. What are the problems that the organization is currently trying to solve?
   b. What are the external factors which are currently of most importance to the organization?
   c. How is the organization financed? How reliable is the funding?
   d. What changes are or have recently taken place within the organization? How many employees reacted to these changes?
   e. How are operations controlled within the organization? What areas require the most control?
   f. How is planning carried out by the organization?
   g. What are the major external factors affecting the organization? At what level of the organization are external contacts made?
   h. What external threats does the organization face? How does it respond to these?
   i. Are there areas in which you believe policies and procedures should be changed? How? Why?
   j. Are employees generally satisfied? Why?
   k. What are the major regulatory concerns of the organization?
   l. How are people within the organization rewarded?
   m. How is the budget developed? Do you think this is appropriate?
4. Journals should be submitted on the second Monday of the month:
   a. February 14
   b. March 13
   c. April 10
   d. May 9
5. *Confidentiality.* The journals are confidential between the student and the faculty supervisor. If it is judged necessary to discuss with the internship preceptor a problem presented in the journal,

the student will be consulted for approval before this is done.

C. Paper. Students will be required to write a paper to include the following:
   1. An assessment of personal strengths and weaknesses.
   2. Evaluation of the applicability of past work experience to future positions.
   3. Long-term goals.
   4. Short-term goals.
   5. Strategies for reaching those goals.

   Further details of this paper will be discussed during seminar. Students with questions should consult the faculty member supervising the internship.

D. Internship Goals and Plan. By February 16, each student, in consultation with his/her preceptor should have developed a set of goals for the internship and a flexible plan. A form is provided for the goals which are to be signed by the preceptor and faculty member.

IV. Evaluation and Grading Methods:

Preceptor's Evaluation	60%
Paper	20%
Journal	20%
	100%

Goals and Objectives for Field Practicum

Student ____________________

____________________ __________
(Signature of Preceptor) Date

____________________ __________
(Signature of University Supervisor) Date

____
(Signature of Student)

Field Visit Form

Student ____________________

Agency ____________________

The following signatures document conferences of the preceptor, faculty supervisor, and student intern.

Date__________

Preceptor ____________________

Faculty Supervisor ____________________

Student Intern ______________________________

Comments:

Date ____________

Preceptor ______________________________

Faculty Supervisor ______________________________

Student Intern ______________________________

Comments:

Evaluation of Student Internship
Health Services Administration

Name of Student ______________________________

Name of Preceptor ______________________________

Place of Internship ______________________________

Address of Facility or Agency ______________________________

Date ______________________________

Evaluation of the student summarized from succeeding pages:

Please circle appropriate letter.

I. Assessment of Knowledge	A	B	C	D	F
II. Skills	A	B	C	D	F
III. Communication Abilities	A	B	C	D	F
IV. Relations with Others	A	B	C	D	F
V. Attitudes	A	B	C	D	F

FINAL GRADE RECOMMENDATION

A Excellent	____
AB Excellent/Good	____
B Good	____
BC Good/Fair	____
C Fair	____
CD Fair/Poor	____
D Poor	____
F Failing	____

Signature of Preceptor ______________________________

I. Assessment of Knowledge
At the conclusion of the internship, the student should be able to:

	Excellent	Good	Fair	Poor	Failing	Not Applicable
1. State the objectives and functions of the agency or facility.	☐	☐	☐	☐	☐	☐
2. Identify the policies and regulations of the facility or agency.	☐	☐	☐	☐	☐	☐
3. Describe the organization of the agency or facility and the relationships among its departments.	☐	☐	☐	☐	☐	☐
4. Discuss the needs and resources of the community.	☐	☐	☐	☐	☐	☐
5. Use networks and linkages within the community.	☐	☐	☐	☐	☐	☐
6. Classify the functions and capabilities of referring and cooperating agencies or organizations and describe how coordination with them is effected.	☐	☐	☐	☐	☐	☐
7. Apply licensure, regulatory and legal requirements.	☐	☐	☐	☐	☐	☐
8. List financing and reimbursement requirements and mechanisms.	☐	☐	☐	☐	☐	☐
9. Pick out the appropriate job descriptions of personnel within the agency or facility.	☐	☐	☐	☐	☐	☐
10. Identify the ways in which control is maintained within the organization.	☐	☐	☐	☐	☐	☐
11. Distinguish a variety of management types and techniques.	☐	☐	☐	☐	☐	☐
12. State the obligations and responsibilities of an administrator.	☐	☐	☐	☐	☐	☐

Grade Recommendation for Knowledge

A Excellent ______
B. Good ______
C Fair ______
D Poor ______
F Failing ______

Comments (Optional)

II. Skills and Professional Competence
At the conclusion of the internship, the student should br able to:

	Excellent	Good	Fair	Poor	Failing	Not Applicable
1. Observe and analyze accurately.	☐	☐	☐	☐	☐	☐

	Excellent	Good	Fair	Poor	Failing	Not Applicable
2. Approach problem-solving in an organized and logical manner.	☐	☐	☐	☐	☐	☐
3. Set reasonable goals.	☐	☐	☐	☐	☐	☐
4. Plan realistically.	☐	☐	☐	☐	☐	☐
5. Implement plans effectively.	☐	☐	☐	☐	☐	☐
6. Work independently.	☐	☐	☐	☐	☐	☐
7. Allocate time well.	☐	☐	☐	☐	☐	☐
8. Make appropriate decisions.	☐	☐	☐	☐	☐	☐
9. Evaluate his/her own work and that of others.	☐	☐	☐	☐	☐	☐

Grade Recommendation for Skills and Professional Competence

A Excellent _____
B Good _____
C Fair _____
D Poor _____
F Failing _____

Comments (Optional)

III. Communication Abilities

At the conclusion of the internship, the student should be able to:

	Excellent	Good	Fair	Poor	Failing	Not Applicable
1. Communicate effectively both in writing and orally.	☐	☐	☐	☐	☐	☐
2. Listen carefully and make use of the views of others.	☐	☐	☐	☐	☐	☐
3. Interact appropriately with clients or patients, employees, providers of services, physicians or consultants and the community at large.	☐	☐	☐	☐	☐	☐
4. Respect the confidentiality of patients or clients and staff.	☐	☐	☐	☐	☐	☐
5. Participate willingly and appropriately at meetings.	☐	☐	☐	☐	☐	☐

Grade Recommendation for Communication Abilities

A Excellent _____
B Good _____
C Fair _____
D Poor _____
F Failing _____

Comments (Optional)

IV. Relations with Others

At the conclusion of the internship, the student should be able to:

	Excellent	Good	Fair	Poor	Failing	Not Applicable
1. Identify and respond to the needs of others.	☐	☐	☐	☐	☐	☐
2. Speak easily and pleasantly with people.	☐	☐	☐	☐	☐	☐
3. Make objective and fair assessments of people and situations.	☐	☐	☐	☐	☐	☐
4. Work cooperatively with others.	☐	☐	☐	☐	☐	☐
5. Accept suggestions or criticism.	☐	☐	☐	☐	☐	☐
6. Adapt easily to changing circumstances.	☐	☐	☐	☐	☐	☐
7. Behave appropriately with staff.	☐	☐	☐	☐	☐	☐
8. Behave appropriately with patients or clients.	☐	☐	☐	☐	☐	☐

Grade Recommendation for Relations with Others

A Excellent _____

B Good _____

C Fair _____

D Poor _____

F Failing _____

Comments (Optional)

V. Attitudes

At the conclusion of the internship, the student should be able to:

	Excellent	Good	Fair	Poor	Failing	Not Applicable
1. Present a neat and professional appearance.	☐	☐	☐	☐	☐	☐
2. Perform assigned tasks within stated time limits.	☐	☐	☐	☐	☐	☐
3. Exhibit an appropriate level of self-confidence.	☐	☐	☐	☐	☐	☐
4. Recognize limits of own authority and that of others.	☐	☐	☐	☐	☐	☐
5. Respect the time and views of others.	☐	☐	☐	☐	☐	☐
6. Recognize own deficiencies and work to correct them.	☐	☐	☐	☐	☐	☐
7. Behave pleasantly in the work environment.	☐	☐	☐	☐	☐	☐

Grade Recommendation for Attitudes

A Excellent _____

b Good _____

C Fair _____

D Poor _____

F Failing _____

Comments (Optional)

Please describe any projects which the intern has completed for you and attach a copy of possible.

Please give your assessment of the student's potential as a health services administrator based on his or her personal and professional characteristics.

Do you have any additional comments?

Do you have any suggestions for the improvement of this evaluation form?

Student's Comments

Student's Signature ______________________________

Faculty Supervisor's Signature ______________________________

Evaluation of Administrative Internship

1. In general, how would you rate your experience with the intern assigned to your organization?
   - ☐ Excellent
   - ☐ Good
   - ☐ Fair
   - ☐ Poor

   Explanation (Optional)

2. Was the intern well-matched to you and your organization?
   - ☐ Yes
   - ☐ No

   Explanation (Optional)

3. Did the intern have any special knowledge or skills that were useful to your organization?
   - ☐ Yes
   - ☐ No

   If the answer is yes, please explain

4. Was the intern adequately prepared for his/her placement?
   - ☐ Yes
   - ☐ No

   Explanation (Optional)

5. Did the university faculty provide adequate information and preparation prior to the start of the internship?
   - ☐ Yes
   - ☐ No

   Explanation (Optional)

6. Was the university supervision adequate during the internship?
   - ☐ Yes
   - ☐ No

   Explanation (Optional)

7. How many times would you like the faculty supervisor to visit during the internship? (Two visits were made this semester.)
   - ☐ Two
   - ☐ More than two
   - ☐ Less than two

   Explanation (Optional)

8. Did you consider the internship a drain on your resources or a contribution to your organization? In what way?

9. Do you have any suggestions for improvement of the internship?

Placement Evaluation

1. Did you feel you were placed well?

2. Did you feel you were accepted as part of the organization?

3. Would you have liked more or less supervision?

4. Was the work load too heavy or too light?

5. Was the work assigned to you relevant?

6. Did you feel your preceptor had realistic expectations of you?

7. Was there anything you would have liked changed at your placement?

8. Were you satisfied with your learning experience, and if not, how could it be improved?

9. Did you feel you were fairly evaluated?

10. Were you satisfied with the visits by faculty?

11. Was the faculty supervision adequate and helpful?

12. Please make any other comments which you feel would be helpful.

EVALUATION

Evaluation is an essential part of any educational program as discussed in Chapter 4. Three examples of evaluation instruments used with the internship were already presented.

In this program, every course taught by non-tenured faculty is evaluated. A standard course evaluation instrument is used within the College of Health Professions and the Department Chairperson observes each non-tenured faculty member at least once each semester.

Faculty members often use their own evaluation forms to elicit students' reaction to various aspects of the course. Examples are shown from two of the courses for which syllabuses were previously given, although the Health Planning and Policy one is from a different year. Obviously these forms will need to be changed as the syllabuses change.

Also included in this section is a form which is used to evaluate students' oral presentations. The form is distributed and discussed with students in the first professional course and is used by faculty members whenever an oral presentation is given in class. After the oral presentation faculty reviews the form with the student so that each student knows the areas in which she/he needs to improve.

Finally, graduating seniors are asked to complete an evaluation of the entire program, and this evaluation is based on the objectives which were set out at the beginning of this chapter. As the program has evolved, student views have been extremely helpful and their comments have complemented faculty evaluations.

Readers should remember that these examples are not intended to present a complete program. They are examples of the types of materials which should be utilized by a program which serves the needs of its students, university and community.

Course Evaluation Form

32–411 Health Law and Regulation

It will be helpful if you will honestly answer the following questions. Your answers will be put aside until all grades for the course have been submitted to the registrar. This protects against the chance that I might recognize someone's handwriting.

Evaluation of the instructor is not included here as this is done within the university-run system.

	Excellent	Good	Fair	Poor
I. Textbooks				
Pozgar, *Legal Aspects of Health Care Administration*	☐	☐	☐	☐
Annas, *The Rights of Hospital Patients*	☐	☐	☐	☐
Conservation Law Foundation, *Legal Handbook for Boards of Health*	☐	☐	☐	☐
II. Various Sections of the Course				
Government and Law in General	☐	☐	☐	☐
Federal and State Government	☐	☐	☐	☐
Use of Federal and State documents	☐	☐	☐	☐
Torts	☐	☐	☐	☐
Other Issues: Risk Management, Labor Law, Reproductive Issues, Death and Dying	☐	☐	☐	☐
III. Guest Speakers and Field Trips				
Government Documents, North Campus Library	☐	☐	☐	☐
State House	☐	☐	☐	☐
Boards of Health	☐	☐	☐	☐
Administrative Law	☐	☐	☐	☐
State–Federal Relations	☐	☐	☐	☐

IV. What was your opinion of the two project assignment?

V. Overall, how would you rate this course?

VI. Do you have any other comments about the course or suggestions to improve it? Was there any element of the course to which you would have liked to devote more time?

Oral Presentation Evaluation Form*
Health Services Administration

Student____________________________ Date________________________

Course ____________________________ Topic________________________

Professor____________________________

ACADEMIC CONTENT

1. Choice of Content
   a. Excellent
   b. Too broad
   c. Too narrow
   d. Did not meet requirement

2. Knowledge of Subject
   a. Excellent
   b. Good
   c. Fair
   d. Poor

PRESENTATION

1. Organization
   a. Clear
   b. Disorganized
   c. Not progressive
   d. Fragmented
2. Methods of Presentation
   a. Excellent/Varied
   b. Good
   c. Fair
   d. Poor
3. Supplementary Materials
   a. Varied
   b. Well done
   c. Needed more variety
   d. Needs to use materials
4. Use of Notes
   a. Talked easily without notes
   b. Used note cards nicely
   c. Read entire presentation
   d. Should have referred to notes
5. General Appearance
   a. Neat
   b. Attractive
   c. Professional
   d. Too casual
6. Facial Expression
   a. Good
   b. Warm
   c. Should smile more
   d. Looked scared
7. Body Movement
   a. Remained in the same spot
   b. Stayed behind lectern
   c. Moved around nicely

DELIVERY

1. Speed and Pacing
   a. Natural
   b. Sometimes too fast
   c. Sometimes too slow
   d. Too fast overall
   e. Too slow overall
2. Skill in Phrasing
   a. Excellent
   b. Good
   c. Fair
   d. Needs improvement
3. Gestures
   a. Natural
   b. Overdone
   c. Inadequate
4. Volume
   a. Appropriate
   b. Good
   c. Too loud
   d. Too soft
   e. Varied
5. Enunciation
   a. Words clearly pronounced
   b. A few words inarticulate
   c. Difficult to understand
6. Voice Expression
   a. Excellent/Varied
   b. Good
   c. Fair
   d. Monotone
7. Eye Contact
   a. Included entire audience
   b. Reasonably good
   c. Looked at same place
   d. Never looked up

PERSONAL TRAITS

1. Nervousness
   a. Not apparent
   b. At beginning only
   c. Slight but not distracting
   d. Apparent - distracted audience
2. Enthusiasm
   a. Evident
   b. Average
   c. Marginal
   d. Not evident
   e. Overdone
3. Assurance
   a. Self-confident
   b. Poised
   c. Developing nicely
   d. Needs improvement
4. Rapport with Audience
   a. Excellent/Warm

b. Good
c. Adequate
d. Lack - detracts from presentation

5. Interaction with Audience
   a. Answered questions well
   b. Responses need improvement
   c. Stimulated discussion
   d. Needed more interaction
   e. Interaction not appropriate/not needed

Overall Presentation
a. Excellent
b. Good/nicely done
c. Adequate
d. Needs great deal of improvement

**Adapted from Health Education Major Lesson Evaluation Form developed by Karen Lorentzen, R.N., Ed.D. and Robert Neal, Ed.D.*

Evaluation of H.S.A. Undergraduate Program

The recipient of the B.S. in Health Services Administration will:	PREPARATION					
	Excellent	Good	Fair	Poor	Inadequate	NA
1. Utilize a broad-based body of knowledge to promote the optimal health of the individual obtained from:						
College core curriculum	☐	☐	☐	☐	☐	☐
University core requirements	☐	☐	☐	☐	☐	☐
Major courses	☐	☐	☐	☐	☐	☐
Major-related courses	☐	☐	☐	☐	☐	☐
2. Identify the major interrelated components, elements, and issues which affect the organization and delivery of contemporary health care services in a changing environment.	☐	☐	☐	☐	☐	☐
3. Describe the relationship of sociocultural, ethical and moral influences on the behavior of consumers, professionals and government agencies.	☐	☐	☐	☐	☐	☐
4. Apply knowledge of the factors influencing health care and its delivery including:						
Legal	☐	☐	☐	☐	☐	☐
Fiscal	☐	☐	☐	☐	☐	☐
Legislative	☐	☐	☐	☐	☐	☐
Environmental	☐	☐	☐	☐	☐	☐

5. Apply administrative and management principles and techniques as they relate within organizational structures to:
   - Goal setting ☐☐☐☐☐☐
   - Planning ☐☐☐☐☐☐
   - Implementation ☐☐☐☐☐☐
   - Evaluation ☐☐☐☐☐☐

6. Exhibit entry-level skills in administration and management practice including skills in:
   - Human Relations ☐☐☐☐☐☐
   - Communication ☐☐☐☐☐☐

7. Recognize the need for continued personal and professional growth. ☐☐☐☐☐☐

Please write below anything else that would be helpful for faculty to know about your preparation in the Health Services Program.

Appendix 1

PROFESSIONAL AND HEALTH-RELATED ORGANIZATIONS

Accrediting Commission on Education for Health Services Administration
Suite 503
1911 North Fort Myer Drive
Arlington, Virginia 22209

American Academy of Medical Administrators
Suite 107
2590 E. Devon Avenue
Des Plaines, Illinois 60018

American Association of Homes for the Aging
Suite 770
1050 17th Street, N.W.
Washington, DC 20036

American Association of Hospital Consultants
2341 Jefferson Davis Highway
Arlington, Virginia 22202

American Cancer Society
219 East 42nd Street
New York, New York 10017

American College of Hospital Administrators
840 North Lake Shore Drive
Chicago, Illinois 60611

American College of Medical Group Administrators
4101 E. Louisiana Avenue
Denver, Colorado 80222

American College of Nursing Home Administrators
4650 East-West Highway
Washington, DC 20014

American Health Care Association
1200 15th Street, N.W.
Washington, DC 20005

American Health Planning Association
Suite 700
1601 Connecticut Avenue, N.W.
Washington, DC 20009

American Heart Association
44 East 23rd Street
New York, New York 10010

American Hospital Association
840 North Lake Shore Drive
Chicago, Illinois 60611

American Medical Association
535 North Dearborn Street
Chicago, Illinois 60610

American National Red Cross
17th and D Streets, N.W.
Washington, DC 20006
(contact local chapters for material)

American Nurses Association
10 Columbus Circle
New York, New York 10019

American Public Health Association
1015 15th Street, N.W.
Washington, DC 20005

Association of Mental Health Administrators
Suite 1230
425 13th Street, N.W.
Washington, DC 20004

Association of University Programs in Health Administration
Suite 503
1911 North Fort Myer Drive
Arlington, Virginia 22209

Blue Cross Association
840 North Lake Shore Drive
Chicago, Illinois 60611

Canadian College of Health Service Executives
Suite 805
410 Laurier Avenue, West
Ottawa, Ontario

Canadian Hospital Association
Suite 800
410 Laurier Avenue, West
Ottawa, Ontario

Gerontological Society
1835 K Street, N.W.
Washington, DC 20006

Hogg Foundation for Mental Health
The University of Texas
Austin, Texas 78712

Hospital Financial Management Association
Suite 500
1900 Spring Road
Oak Brook, Illinois 60521

Medical Group Management Association
4101 E. Louisiana Avenue
Denver, Colorado 80222

National Association of Health Services Executives
2231 S. Western Avenue
Los Angeles, California 90018

National Association for Mental Health
10 Columbus Circle
New York, New York 10019

National Coordinating Council on Drug Abuse
P.O. Box 19400
Washington, DC 20036

National Hospice Organization
Suite 402
1901 North Fort Myer Drive
Arlington, Virginia 22209

National League for Nursing
59th Street and Columbus Circle
New York, New York 10019

Pharmaceutical Manufacturers Association
1155 15th Street, N.W.
Washington, DC 20005

Society for Nuclear Medicine
305 East 45th Street
New York, New York 20017

Appendix 2

JOURNALS OF INTEREST

Abstracts of Health Care Management
American Journal of Public Health
Harvard Business Review
Health Affairs
Health Care Financing Review
Health Services Research
Hospital and Health Services Administration
Hospital and Community Psychiatry
Hospitals
Inquiry
International Journal of Health Services
JAMA: Journal of the American Medical Association
Journal of Ambulatory Care Management
Journal of Gerontology
Journal of Health and Social Behavior
Journal of Health, Politics, Policy and Law
Journal of Long-Term Care Administration
Medical Care
Milbank Memorial Fund Quarterly, Health and Society
New England Journal of Medicine
Social Security Bulletin
Topics in Health Care Financing
Trustee
Urban Health
Washington Report on Medicine and Health

Bibliography

1. Accrediting Commission on Education for Health Services Administration: The Accreditation Process and the Use of the Survey Questionnaire, 1982.
2. Aquilina D: Toward Competition in Boston's Health Care Market: A Health Care Task Force Report on the Status of HMOs in Boston, Massachusetts. Business Round Table, 1982.
3. Association of University Programs in Health Administration: *Guidelines for a Clinical/Administrator-in-Training Experience in a Long-Term-Care Facility.* Washington, DC, n.d.
4. Bellin LE, Weeks LE: *The Challenge of Administering Health Services: Career Pathways.* Washington: AUPHA, 1981.
5. Boissoneau R: *Continuing Education in the Health Professions.* Rockville: Aspen, 1980.
6. Borus ME, Buntz GC, Tash WR: *Evaluating the Impact of Health Programs: A Primer.* Cambridge: MIT, 1982.
7. Boyles MV, Morgan MK, McCaulley MH: *The Health Professions.* Philadelphia: Saunders, 1982.
8. Bruess CD, Gay JE: *Implementing Comprehensive School Health.* New York: Macmillan, 1978.
9. Campbell OT, Stanley JC: *Experimental and Quasi-Experimental Designs for Research.* Chicago: Rand McNally, 1963.
10. Campion EW, Bang A, May MI: Why Acute Care Hospitals Must Undertake Long-Term Care. *N Engl J Med, 308:*71-75, 1983.
11. Charns MP, Schaefer MJ: *Health Care Organizations: A Model for Management.* Englewood Cliffs: Prentice Hall, 1983.
12. Commission on Education ofr Health Administration: *Education for Health Administration,* 1. Ann Arbor: Health Administration Press, 1975.
13. Crichton A, Neuhauser D, eds: *The New Epidemiology.* Arlington, VA: AUPHA, 1982.
14. Curtis JD, Papenfuss RL: *Health Instruction A Task Approach.* Minneapolis: Burgess, 1980.
15. Dever GEA: *Community Health Analysis: A Holistic Approach.* Rockville: Aspen, 1980.
16. Elpers J, Corwell A: How Many Beds? An Overview of Resource Planning. *Hosp and Com Psychiatry 33:*755-761, 1982.
17. Enthoven AC: Consumer-Centered vs. Job-Centered Health Insurance. *Harvard Business Review, 57:*141-147, 1979.

18. Enthoven AC: Consumer Choice Health Plan. *N Engl J Med, 298:*650-658, 1978.
19. Fodor JT, Dalis GT: *Health Instruction: Theory and Application,* 3. Philadelphia: Lea and Febiger, 1981.
20. Ford CW, Morgan MK: *Teaching in the Health Professions.* St. Louis: CV Mosby, 1976.
21. Gali N: *Foundation and Principles of Health Education.* New York: Wiley, 1978.
22. Georgopolous BS: The Hospital as an Organization and Problem-Solving System. Georgopolous BS, ed. *Organization Research on Health Institutions.* Ann Arbor: Institute for Social Research, 1972.
23. Gibson RM, Wlado DR: National Health Expenditures, 1981. *Health Care Financing Review, 2:*1-36, 1982.
24. Green LW, Kreuter MW, Deeds SG, Partridge KB: *Health Education Planning A Diagnostic Approach.* Palo Alto: Mayfield, 1980.
25. Haiman T: *Supervisory Management for Health Care and Institutions.* St. Louis: Catholic Health Administration, 1973.
26. Health Systems Agency of New York: Phase II MFRC. New York, November, 1982.
27. Hershey N: *Hospital-Physician Relationships. Case Studies and Commentaries on Medical Staff Problems.* Rockville: Aspen, 1982.
28. Herzberg F, Mausner B, Snyderman B: *The Motivation to Work.* New York: John Wiley, 1959.
29. Hodgetts RM, Cascio CM: *Modern Health Care Administration.* New York: Academic, 1983.
30. Kaluzny AD, Warner DM, Warren DG, Zelman WN: *Management of Health Services.* Englewood Cliffs: Prentice Hall, 1982.
31. Levey S, Loomba NP: *Health Care Administration.* Philadelphia: Lippincott, 1973.
32. Maslow AH: *Motivation and Personality,* 2. New York: Harper & Row, 1970.
33. McClelland DH: *The Achieving Society.* New York: Van Nostrand Reinhold, 1961.
34. McConnel CR: *The Health Care Supervisor's Casebook.* Rockville: Aspen, 1982.
35. Metzger N: *Personnel Administration in the Health Services Industry,* 2. New York: Spectrum, 1979.
36. Osterling RD, ed: *Guidelines for Conducting an Administrator-in-Training Program.* Austin: National Association of Boards of Examiners for Nursing Home Administrators, 1981.
37. P.L. 93-641, National Health Planning and Resources Development Act, January 4, 1975, 93rd Congress.
38. Pressman J, Wildavsky A: *Implementation: How Great Expectations in Washington are Dashed in Oakland.* Berkeley: University of California, 1973.

39. Rakich JS, Longest BB, Darr K: *Cases in Health Services Management.* Philadelphia: Saunders, 1983.
40. Rakich JS, Longest BB, O'Donovan TR: *Managing Health Care Organizations.* Philadelphia: Saunders, 1977.
41. Sager A: Urban Voluntary Hospitals: Predictable Closure Relocation Patterns. *Hospital Prog, 62:*45-63, 1981.
42. Scott GW, Carlo MW: *On Becoming a Health Educator*, 2. Dubuque: Brown, 1974.
43. Simon HA: *Administrative Behavior: A Study of Decision-Making Process in Administrative Organization.* New York: Macmillan, 1961.
44. Simon HA: *The New Science of Management.* Englewood Cliffs: Prentice Hall, 1960.
45. Stoner JAF: *Management.* Englewood Cliffs: Prentice Hall, 1978.
46. Thompson F: *Health Policy and the Bureaucracy: Politics and Implementation.* Cambridge: MIT, 1981.
47. Tourigny AW, LaFrance SV: *Baccalaureate Health Administration Graduates: A Decade Review.* Washington, DC: Association of University Programs in Health Administration, 1983.
48. Veninga RL: *The Human Side of Health Administration. A Guide for Hospital, Nursing and Public Health Administrators.* Englewood Cliffs: Prentice Hall, 1982.
49. Warner DM, Holloway OC: *Decision Making and Control for Health Administration: The Management of Quantitative Analysis.* Ann Arbor: Health Administration Press, 1978.
50. Warner K, Luce BR: *Cost Benefit and Cost Effectiveness Analysis in Health Care: Principles and Potential.* Ann Arbor: Health Administration Press, 1982.
51. Weiss C: *Evaluation Research: Methods of Assessing Program Effectiveness.* Englewood Cliffs: Prentice Hall, 1972.
52. Willgoose CE: *Health Teaching in Secondary Schools*, 3. New York: Saunders, 1982.
53. Wilson FA, Neuhauser D: *Health Services in the United States*, 2. Cambridge: Ballinger, 1982.
54. Zelman WN, Vraciu RA, Kahn CN, eds: *Health Care Finanical Management: Curriculum Objectives and Bibliography.* Arlington, VA: AUPHA, 1983.

Index